INDEX & REPERTORY
TO THE
HOMŒOPATHIC
DRUG PICTURES

OF DR M. L. TYLER

INDEX & REPERTORY TO THE HOMŒOPATHIC DRUG PICTURES

OF DR M. L. TYLER

BY

N. W. JOLLYMAN

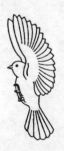

SAFFRON WALDEN
THE C. W. DANIEL COMPANY LIMITED

First Published in 1988
by The C. W. Daniel Company Ltd
1 Church Path, Saffron Walden,
Essex, CB10 1JP, England

ISBN 0 85207 201 5

Design and Production in association
with Book Production Consultants, Cambridge
Typeset by Cambridge Photosetting Services
Printed in Great Britain by Biddles Ltd, Guildford

CONTENTS

Preface   7
Remedies & their abbreviations   11
Index and repertory   13
Bibliography   222

PREFACE

Students of Homoeopathy have long been intrigued, enlightened and entertained by the superb analyses Dr. Tyler has given in her HOMŒOPATHIC DRUG PICTURES of the relationships between the symptomatic 'pictures' of drugs and the picture presented by a person who is suffering from ill-health in one way or another.

In considering the appropriate remedy for a patient I often realised that Dr. Tyler had in fact covered similar cases but there was no easy way of remembering where, in her long book, reference had been made to similar circumstances.

This Index and Repertory was therefore born partly out of frustration and partly as a tribute in recognition of the brilliant insight Dr. Tyler had of the PERSONALITIES of the remedies which she has written about. She shows how each differs from the others in some vital aspect – in the same way that human personalities differ.

Dr. Tyler emphasizes over and over again the necessity of prescribing a remedy ONLY IF THE SYMPTOMS AGREE. It is quite apparent from her anecdotes that a remedy may be prescribed on the strength of a particular symptom even though that remedy had not, up to then, been considered suitable for that kind of ailment. These are very telling descriptions of prescribing for the PATIENT and not the complaint.

The wealth of information in the Drug Pictures cannot be found anywhere else and goes beyond the scope of any one Materia Medica in UNDERSTANDING the remedies. The Materia Medica will of course still have to be consulted for the minutae of other symptoms not included here and of course for remedies which have not been included in the book.

Although necessarily in alphabetical order, I have tried to set out the information in such a way that it is readily comparable with information in the Materia Medica. The Index can in fact be used as a mini-Repertory to point the way in which one should go. I have taken certain liberties with words and have tried to simplify references so the actual wording in the Index may be slightly different from that of the original text – e.g. 'frequent' pulse comes under the reference for 'rapid' pulse; 'unquenchable' thirst will be found under 'excessive' thirst.

Some knowledge of anatomy is presumed. e.g. information on 'fontanelles' will be found under 'HEAD', 'Canthi' under EYES etc. This makes it more possible to group similarities under symptoms in the same manner as used in homoeopathic Materia Medica.

Hahnemann's name appears so frequently I did not think it would be helpful to add him to the Index, except where his books are specifically mentioned.

To speed up the process of checking suitable remedies I have shown, where appropriate, the name of the remedy as well as the page reference. This has the added advantage of highlighting certain remedies which appear more than once under a specific heading.

Where two or more remedies are mentioned by Tyler against a particular symptom these are included, together with the remedy and page on which they are mentioned. Where a remedy's name is given without a page number it will be found on the page referred to against the NEXT remedy. e.g. Chronic headaches. Nat. mur., (Bry. 147) If there are brackets round the next remedy it means that comment on that particular symptom has been made on that page, but the remedy mentioned may not be suitable for that symptom. If however NO brackets are given then both, or more, remedies are applicable.

I wished to include certain important ideas which did not appear to come under any one particular heading. I have therefore lumped them together under a descriptive heading and I suggest an initial look through the Index will give the reader an insight into how best to use it. e.g. 'First aid' covers such well known concepts as 'air hunger' and 'corpse reviver' which would be difficult to list under any other heading.

Occasionally I have underlined a remedy where it is apparent that it is an outstanding remedy for that symptom and may be deemed to be a 'specific' Dr. Tyler discusses specifics on page 547.

Sometimes there may appear to be duplication of a reference, perhaps one remedy is mentioned under the heading of another, as well as in its own right. This has been done deliberately as in many instances connections are made between two or more remedies and it is these connections, similarities or exceptions which are the true value of Dr. Tyler's writings.

The repertory should NOT be taken as a complete one for any remedy, or even for any symptom, but is a guide to those remedies which are most likely to be useful in considering a particular symptom. The normal repertories and Materica Medica should also be used.

To make things easier for the non-medically trained reader I have included a short explanation of the more unusual and often slightly outdated words mentioned in the text. Fuller definitions may be required in which case a medical Dictionary will be found useful. In this connection I have to admit defeat over the word 'Ecptysis' mentioned on page 542 and this may be a misprint in the original text.

Dr. Tyler mentions on page 783 that "the less a physician knows of Materia Medica, the oftener he gives Sulphur". An understanding of the 125 remedies covered by Dr. Tyler will ensure that the above remark cannot be levelled at anyone who studies her delightful descriptions of these major remedies.

N. W. Jollyman.
Elton, Peterborough
1987

9

Remedies and their abbreviations

Abrotanum.	Abrot	Coffea cruda.	Coffea
Aconitum.	Acon.	Colchicum autumnale	Colch.
Aesculus hippocastanum.	Aesc.	Collinsonia canadensis.	Collin.
Aethusa cynapium.	Aeth.	Colocynth.	Coloc.
Agaricus muscarius.	Agar.	Conium maculatum.	Con.
Ailanthus glandulosa.	Ail.	Crotalus horridus.	Crot.
Allium cepa	Allium	Cuprum.	Cup.
Alumina.	Alum.	Cyclamen.	Cycl.
Ammonium carbonicum.	Ammon. carb.	Drosera.	Dros.
		Dulcamara.	Dulc.
Anacardium crudum.	Anac.	Ferrum.	Ferr.
Antimonium tartaricum.	Ant. tart.	Ferrum phosphoricum.	Ferr. phos.
Apis	Apis	Gelsemium.	Gels.
Argentum nitricum	Arg. nit.	Glonoine.	Glon.
Arnica montana	Arn.	Graphites.	Graph.
Arsenicum.	Ars.	Hepar sulphuris.	Hepar.
Asafoetida.	Asaf.	Hyoscyamus niger.	Hyos.
Aurum.	Aur.	Hypericum.	Hyp.
Baptisia tinctoria.	Bapt.	Ignatia.	Ign.
Belladonna.	Bell.	Iodum.	Iod.
Bellis perennis.	Bellis	Ipecacuanha.	Ipec.
Borax.	Borax.	Iris versicolor.	Iris.
Bromium.	Brom.	Kali bichromicum.	Kali bich.
Bryonia.	Bry.	Kali bromatum.	Kali br.
Calcarea carbonica.	Calc. c.	Kali carbonicum.	Kali carb.
Calcarea phosphorica.	Calc. p.	Kali sulphuricum.	Kali s.
Calcarea sulphurica.	Calc. s.	Kreosotum.	Kreos.
Camphora.	Camph.	Lac caninum.	Lac. can.
Cannabis indica.	Cann.	Lachesis.	Lach.
Cantharis.	Canth.	Ledum palustre.	Led.
Capsicum.	Caps.	Lilium tigrinum.	Lil. tig
Carbo vegetabilis.	Carbo v.	Lycopodium.	Lyc.
Caulophyllum.	Caul.	Magnesia phosphorica.	Mag. phos.
Causticum.	Caust.	Medorrhinum.	Med.
Ceanothus americanus.	Cean.	Muriatic acid.	Mur. ac.
Chamomilla.	Cham.	Natrum muriaticum.	Nat. mur.
Chelidonum majus.	Chel.	Natrum phosphoricum.	Nat. phos.
China.	China.	Natrum sulphuricum.	Nat. sul.
Cistus canadensis.	Cistus	Nitric acid	Nit. ac.
Cocculus.	Cocc.	Nux moschata.	Nux mosch.

Nux vomica.	Nux v.	Salicylic acid.	Sal. ac.
Opium.	Opium.	Sanguinaria çanadensis.	Sang.
Ornithogalum umbellatum.	Ornith.	Sanicula aqua.	San.
Paeonia	Paeonia.	Sepia.	Sep.
Palladium.	Pall.	Silica.	Sil.
Petroleum, Oleum petre.	Pet.	Staphisagria.	Staph.
Phosphoric acid.	Phos. ac.	Stramonium.	Stram.
Phytolacca decandra.	Phyt.	Sulphur.	Sul.
Picric acid.	Pic. ac.	Symphitum.	Symph.
Platinum.	Plat.	Tarentula	Tarent.
Plumbum.	Plumb	Terebinthina.	Tereb.
Psorinum.	PSor.	Theridion.	Ther.
Ptelia trifoliata	Ptelia	Thuja occidentalis.	Thuja
Pulsatilla.	Puls.	Tuberculinum.	Tub.
Pyrogenium	Pyrogen.	Urtica urens.	Urtica.
Ranunculus bulbosus.	Ran. b.	Veratrum album.	Ver. alb.
Ranunculus sceleratus.	Ran. sc.	Veratrum viride.	Ver. vir.
Rhododendron.	Rhod.	Viburnum opulus.	Vib.
Rhus Toxicodendron.	Rhus.	Viscum album.	Viscum.
Ruta graveolens.	Ruta		

INDEX & REPERTORY

A

ABDOMEN
PAIN:

burning Acon. *10*, Ars. *95*, Caps. *199. 201.* Cicuta *262*, Graph *399.* Kreos. *481.* Tereb. *810* Sul *782.*

intense. Ars. *97, 99.* Colch. *302.*

violent. Ant. tart. *66.* Coloc. *315.*

shooting. Ign. *430.*

stitching. Kali carb. *472.*

< motion. Kali carb *472.*

sticking, shooting, < motion. Bry. *143.*

cutting. Caps *201.* Hyos. *414.* Kali carb. *472.*

long lasting. Bell. *122.*

excessive. Plumbum *668.*

paroxysmal. Coloc *316. 319.*

spasmodic like gallstones. Kali bich. *460.*

soreness above pelvis. Ver. vir. *861.*

pain after discharging flatus. Puls. *684.*

tensive, in hypogastrium. Aur *110.* Caps. *201,* Cimic *272.*

in umbilical region. Coloc. *318,* Iris. *452.* Mur. ac. *565.* Staph. *763.*

in upper abdomen. Graph. *399.*

in front of abdomen. Ipec. *445.*

in lower abdomen. Vib. *864.*

in umbilicus. Dulc. *364, 366,* Ipec. *441. 444/5* Nat. sul. *585.* Ptelea *680,* Plumbum *668.*

radiating to other parts. Plumbum *668,* Pyrogen *691.*

colicky before menses. Kali carb. *473.*

> hard pressure. Coloc *316.*

MYALGIA (PAIN IN MUSCLES) OF DIAPHRAGM.
Cimic *271, 275.*

CONSTRICTION AND TENSION IN:

epigastrium. Tarent *800.*

pit of stomach. Cimic. *273.*

right hypochondrium. Chel. *250.*

both hypochondria. Ipec. *445.*

hepatic region. Lyc. *518.*

HARD, TENSE.
Silica. *753.*

13

CONSTANT COLIC IN . . .
Tereb. *812.*

ABDOMINAL WALL:
tingling. Calc. p. *168.*
numb and aching. Calc. p. *168.*

PULSATIONS OF ARTERIES
IN . . .
Caps. *203.*

SPASMS IN . . .
Cocc. *291.*

EXCESSIVE CRAMPS IN . . .
Cuprum, Ver. alb. *857,* Vib.
864.

SPASMODIC INTERNAL HEAVING
IN EPIGASTRIUM.
Cocc. *298,* Crocus, Thuja,
Cycl. *351.*

METEORISM.
Acon. *10,* Ars. *99,* Asaf *101,*
Bapt. *112.* Calc *159. 161.* Carbo
v. *211,* Cham. *240.* Colch. *304,*
309., Cicuta *263,* Cocc. *292, 296.*
Lyc. *518,* Med. *535.* Nux
mosch. *599,* Nux v. *605,* Tereb
811.
excessive. Asaf. *103,* China *260,*
Colch. *304,* Coloc *318.*
> from flatus. Lyc. *518.*
after normal meal. China.
(Lyc. *521*).
after eating a little. Lyc. *521.*
must loosen clothes. Lyc.,
Mag. phos. *525.*
swollen, with emaciation in
rest of body: Bar. c., Sil., Nat.
mur. Sul. Calc. Iod. Abrot. *3*
emaciation everywhere except
abdomen. Calc. *161.*

FLATULENCE AND GURGLING ON
R. SIDE. Calc. *161,* Caps.
201.
in upper abdomen. Puls
684.

RUMBLING:
in right ileo-caecal region.
Nat. sul. *583.*
in whole abdomen. Nat. sul.
585, Phos ac. *638,* Nitric ac. *591*
San *734,* Sepia *741.* Sul. *788.*
> by eating. Graph. Mosch.
Sul. San. *734.*
loud. Ant. crud. *55,* Aur *110,*
Lyc. *518.*

GRIPING AND PINCHING:
Coloc *319,* Coloc. Vib. Bell.
(Ferr. phos *375*).

EXCESSIVE TENDERNESS.
Bell. *122.*

ASCITES.
Colch. *309,* Apis. *71.* Ars. *94.*
Lyc. *518,* Med. *535,* Tereb. *812.*
with anasarca. Tereb. *812.*

MUSCLES SORE.
Batp. *115,* Cimic *272,* Pyrogen
691.

SENSITIVE.
Acon. *10.*

< JUST BELOW NAVEL.
Coloc *319.*

COLD.
Aeth. 20. Kreos *480.*

NAVEL:
sensation of drawing pains
in . . . Plat. *660,* Plumb *664.*
retraction of . . . Plumbum,
663, 668.

14

as if navel attached to spine.
Plat. Plumb *663/4. 668. 670.*

sore. Kali c. Nat. mur. (Calc.
161). Iris *452* Coloc. *318*. Phos.
ac. *638*.

PRESSURE IN EPIGASTRIUM.
Nux. v. *605*.

FERMENTATION IN
EPIGASTRIUM.
Plat. *661*.

INCARCERATED OR
STRANGULATED HERNIA.
Plumbum. *666*.

TYMPANITES:
as result of decomposition of
food. Carbo. v. (Cocc. *292*).

as result of retention of flatus.
Cocc. *292*. Rhus. *716*. Tereb.
811. Ail. *28*.

with shreddy, watery, bloody
stools. Colch. *304*.

METASTASIS FROM GOUT.
Colch. *309*.

FEELS HOLLOW.
Cocc. *298*.

FEELS HEAVY.
Graph. *399*.

< SITTING AND < STOOPING.
Coloc. Ant. tart. *69*.

FEELS FULL OF FLATUS.
Graph. *399*. Staph. *763*.

INTESTINES:
sundry diseases with cold
sweat on forehead. Veratrum.
Ant. tart. *62*.

sundry diseases with
drowsiness. Ant. tart. *62*.

ENTERITIS.
Ant. tart. *68*.

SENSATION:
as if everything in abdomen
would burst. Caps. *201*. Nitric
ac. *593*.

as if everything would burst
through the mouth. Asaf. *103*.
105.

as if intestines were drawn
towards the spine. Plumbum,
Plat. Tereb. *812*.

of 'goneness'. Lyc. Sep. Ptelea.
680, Sepia. *741*. Tub. *837*, Phos.
642. Sul. *788*. Phos. *645*.

of 'goneness' with burning
sensation between shoulder
blades. Phos. *642*.

as if constricted as if by a
string. Chel. *250*, Plat. *660*.

as if sharp stones rubbed
against each other in
abdomen. Cocc. *298*.

as if abdomen were full of
stones. Ant. tart. Calc. *161*.

as of something alive in . . .
Calc. p. *168*, Cycl. *351*. Thuja.
829. Crocus, Thuja. Sepia. *743*.

as if an animal were wriggling
in epigastrium. Chel. *250*.

as if something moved up and
down. Crocus. Thuja. Sanic.
Lyc. *518*.

as of reversed peristalsis. Asaf.
103.

of weakness in abdominal ring.
Nux. v. *605*.

CHILDREN WITH SUNKEN
FLABBY ABDOMEN.
Calc. p. *165/6*.

FEELS STUFFED AFTER A MEAL
AND MUST LOOSEN CLOTHING.
Lyc. San. *734*.

DIGESTIVE SYMPTOMS HAVE
SYMPATHETIC PAIN IN HEAD,
FACE AND TEETH.
Tarent *800*.

ABORTION

THREATENED, FROM FALLS,
SHOCK ETC.
Arnica. *89, 91*.

THREATENED.
Caul *216, 217*, Cimic *274*. Ipec.
441.

IMPENDING.
Kali carb. *473*. Nux. mosch.
597.

FROM WEAKNESS.
Caul *291*.

WITH BLACK NON-COAGULABLE
BLOOD.
Crot. *338*.

ABSCESS

OF ANY KIND.
Bell *125*, Sil. *759*.

CHRONIC.
Stram. *772*.

WITH SEVERE PAIN.
Ars. Anthracinum. Tarent.
807.

WITH SWELLING.
Hyp. *420*.

WITH BLUISH COLOUR.
Tarent. cub. *805*.

WITH BURNING PAINS.
Tarent cub. *805*.

WITH DARK UNCOAGULABLE
BLOOD.
Lach. Crot. *333*.

WITH CEASELESS MOVEMENT.
Pyrogen. (Crot. *334*).

WITH INCOORDINATION
BETWEEN PULSE AND
TEMPERATURE.
Pyrogen (Crot. *334*).

PALMAR ABSCESS WITH HIGH
FEVER.
Crot. *333*.

AXILLARY ABSCESSES.
Tarent. (Crot. *334*).

BELOW COCCYX.
Paeonia. *624*.

IN MOUTH.
Pyrogen. *694*.

> COLD.
Ledum. *500/1*, Lyc. *521*.

> heat.
Ars. (Ledum. *501*).

RESULT OF INSECT STINGS.
Tarent. (Crot. *334*).

ACIDOSIS
Nat. mur. *576/7*.

ACTINOMYCOSIS
"RAY FUNGUS" — CHRONIC
SUPPURATIVE DISEASE OF
THE MOUTH WITH ABSCESSES
AND LATER ULCERS.
Nitric. ac. *589*.

ADIPSIA
ABSENCE OF THIRST.
  Puls. *681, 684*, Staph. *763*.

ADDISON'S DISEASE
  Calc. *159*.

ADYNAMIA
GREAT DEPRESSION OF VITAL
  FORCE.
  Tub. *839*.

AGGLUTININ
  Bapt. *111*.

AGUE
  Ars. *95*, Caps. *109*. Cean. *234*,
  China. *254*. Ipec. *440* Nat. mur.
  569, Nat. sul. *583*.

ALBUMEN
  Calc. p. *169*.

ALBUMINARIA
PRESENCE OF ALBUMEN IN
  URINE. see URINE.

ALUMINIUM
ANTIDOTE TO POISONING BY . . .
  Alum. *35, 40*.

ALUMINOPHOBIA FEAR OF
  POSSIBLE ALUMINIUM
  POISONING.
  Alum. *33*.

AMAUROSIS
LOSS OF SIGHT DUE TO DISEASE
  OTHER THAN IN THE EYE.
  Plumbum *666*.

AMENORRHEA
ABSENCE OF MENSTRUAL FLOW
  DURING THE TIME OF LIFE
  WHEN IT SHOULD APPEAR.
  see FEMALE SEX.

AMBLYOPIA
DEFECTIVE VISION FOR WHICH
  NO RECOGNISABLE CAUSE
  EXISTS IN ANY PART OF THE
  EYE. see EYES.

ANAEMIA
  Nat. mur. (Ferr. *373*). China.
  Ferr. phos. *381*.

PERNICIOUS.
  Calc. *155*, Picric ac. *657*.

CHLOROTIC.
  Calc. *156*. *Calc. p. 169*. Ferr.
  371.

CEREBRAL.
  Borax. *133*.

FROM HAEMORRHAGES.
  Ferr. *371*.

FROM EXHAUSTING DISEASES.
  Ferr. *371*.

WITH SUDDEN FIERY FLUSHING
  OF FACE.
  Ferr. *373*.

WITH THROBBING ALL
  THROUGH THE BODY.
  Kali. carb. *471*.

WITH GREAT DEBILITY.
  Kali. carb. *474*.

WITH PALE MUCOUS
  MEMBRANES.
  Ferr. *373*, Graph. *397*.

17

WITH ANAEMIC LOOK.
Calc. p. *165*.

ESPECIALLY IN YOUNG GIRLS.
Alum. *39*.

WEARY BREATHLESS.
Calc. *154*.

FROM LEAD IN WATER.
Alumina. *33*.

FROM RAPID REDUCTION IN
NUMBER OF RED CORPUSCLES.
Plumbum *668/9*.

DROPSY AFTER LOSS OF BLOOD
CAUSING ANAEMIA.
China 260.

ANALGESICS
Bell *117*.

ANASARCA
GENERAL DROPSY.
Tereb *812*.

ANEURISM
DILATION OF ARTERY. see
VEINS.

ANOREXIA
IMMEDIATELY SATIATED ON
EATING A LITTLE.
Cycl. *350*.

THROUGH EXTREME DISLIKE TO
ALL FOOD.
Ferr. *370*.

ANTHRAX
Ars. *98*.

ANTHROPOPHOBIA
MISTRUST OF OTHERS. see
MENTALS.

ANTIDOTES
POISON ANTIDOTED BY ITS
POTENCIES.
Alum. *35*, Coffea *300*.

ANTI-PSORICS
Sulc. Calc. Lyc. *520*. Ammon.
carb. *45*.

ANXIOUS. ANXIETY
see WORRY.

APHONIA
FAILURE OF VOICE. see
THROAT.

APHTHAE
Sul. *788*.

INFLAMED.
Aeth. *20*, Merc. *542*.

IN MOUTH.
Mur. ac. *564*.

FETID, SOUR SMELLING.
Mur. ac. *564*.

APOPLEXY
Ant. crud. *56*, Opium. *612*.

THREATENED.
Coffea. *300*.

FEAR OF.
Ferr. *371*..

WITH HIGH BLOOD PRESSURE.
Opium. Glon. *394*.

APPENDICITIS
Bell. *117*.

APPETITE
Sul. *788*, Iod. *432, 433*. Med. *531*. Plat. *662*.

LOSS OF APPETITE.
Abrot. *2*. Allium *30*. Ant. crud. *52*. Med. *531*. Calc. *161*. Chel. *250*, Cocc. *296*. Colch. *302*. Ipec. *445*, Kali bich. *458*. Mez. *553*.

LITTLE OR NO APPETITE.
Cycl. *350*. Puls. (Iod. *436*).

LITTLE BUT DESIRE TO EAT.
Mez. *546*.

POOR.
Picric ac. *656*. Ptelea. *679*, Puls. *686*. Sil. *751*.

REPUGNANCE TO FOOD AND DRINK.
Cocc. *291*, Cycl. *350*. Ferr. *372*.

LACK OF FOOD LEADS TO HEADACHES.
Sul. *788*.

GREAT APPETITE.
Psor *676*, Abrot. *2*. Colch. *308*, Lac. can. *488*.

RAVENOUS.
Cann. *183*. Cina. *280/1*. Iod. *432, 436*. Lyc. *517*.

RAVENOUS, WHILE EMACIATING.
Abrot. *2*. Iod. *436*.

CANINE HUNGER.
Ferr. *370*, Sul. *788*.

NOON AND EVENING.
Mez. *553*.

ALTERNATING WITH LOSS OF APPETITE.
Iod *433*. Ferr. *370*.

FEELS FULL, YET STILL HUNGRY.
Lyc. *515, 517*.

HUNGRY WHEN WAKING AT NIGHT.
Lyc. *519*.

CONSTANT HUNGER – WITH DIARRHOEA.
Pet. *631*.

ONLY FEELS WELL WHILE EATING.
Iod. 435.

ONLY FEELS WELL AFTER EATING.
Iod. *432*, Mez. *546*.

GNAWING SENSATION IN THE STOMACH.
Cina. *283*. Sepia *747*.

GREAT HUNGER AFTER A MEAL.
Cina. *283*, Lac. can. *488*.

GNAWING HUNGER, SELDOM SATISFIED.
Sepia. *747*.

GNAWING HUNGER, WITH PROLAPSUS.
Sepia. 747.

EXTREME HUNGER EVEN WHILE STOMACH IS FULL OF FOOD.
Staph. *766*.

HUNGER I I. A.M.
Sul. *790*.

HUNGER WITH INTENSE THIRST.
Tarent *780*. Ver. alb. *854*.

FULL AND BLOATED AFTER
EATING.
Lyc. *517*.

WITH METALLIC TASTE.
Cocc. *296*.

HUNGER WITHOUT APPETITE.
Rhus. *711*, Sang. *731*.

COMPLAINTS > EATING.
Sepia *747*.

WITH HICCOUGH.
Chel *250*.

ARBORVITAL
REMEDIES.
Ornithogalum. *617, 621*.

ARGYRIA
DUSKY SKIN AS RESULT OF
TAKING SILVER SALTS OVER A
LONG PERIOD.
Arg. nit. *77*.

ARMS
PAIN:
down arm. Cimic *273*. Cycl.
350, Staph. *764*.

pain in joint of humerus. Ign.
431.

Violent pain. < lying still.
Rhus *713*.

pain as from a blow in elbow
joint. Ruta *721*.

rheumatic pain in . . . Sang.
729.

cramping pain in Left upper
arm. Cina. *283*.

numbness and paralytic
feelings. Cocc *297*, Graph. *400*
Nat. mur. *574*.

Paralytic pain in . . . Colch.
308, Cycl. *350*.

paralytic pain extending down
to fingers. Staph. *764*.

making it difficult to write.
Cycl. *350*.

WRISTS:
sprained. Ruta *717*.

sore, as if bruised. Ruta *721*.

sensation of sprained wrist.
Rhod. *741*. Rhus. *713*.

inflamed. Abrot *2*.

rheumatic. Ruta. Abrot *2*.

pain in . . . Ammon carb. *42*.

possible writer's cramp. Cycl.
349.

GRASPING SENSATION IN UPPER
ARM.
Nux. mosch. *598*.

STITCHES IN . . .
Cocc. *297*.

'FALL ASLEEP'
Cocc. *292*.

'WRIST DROP' AS RESULT OF
LEAD POISONING.
Plumbum *665*.

APPEAR TO GO TO SLEEP ON
GRASPING ANYTHING.
Cham. *241*.

APPEAR TO WEIGH
HUNDREDWEIGHT.
Ammon. carb. *43*.

SPASM IN RIGHT ARM.
Amon. carb. *43*.

ITCHING IN UPPER ARM.
Ruta *721*.

ARNOT-SCHULTZ LAW
Opium *615*, Thuja. *828*.

ARTHRITIS
PAIN:

in joints. Colch. *305*, Dros. *359*,
Iod. *433*. Med. *532*.

in small joints. Colch. *305*,
Dros. *359*, Med. *532*.

in periosteum. Colch. *305*.

in ankles and feet. Dros *359*.

in long bones. Caust. *223*.

in hands and feet. Caul *220*.

< at night. Cimic. *274*.

< in wet weather. Cimic *274*.

< in wet damp weather. Nat.
sul. *582*.

RHEUMATOID ARTHRITIS:

Puls. *682*. Nat. phos. *577*. *Ant.
crud* (almost specific) *58*.

beginning at the menopause.
Caul. *220*.

< during periods. Caul. *220*.

chronic. Phyt. *653*, Sepia *746*,
Iod. *433*. Nat. sul. *582*.

gonorrheal in origin. Thuja
824.

tuberculous in origin. Tub *832*.

arthritic nodes. Rhod. *704*.

with tuberculous family history.
Tub. bov. Caust. Dros. *359*.

ASCARIDES
ROUNDWORMS.

Calc. *161*, Ign. *425*.

ASCITES
DROPSICAL SWELLING OF THE
ABDOMEN. see ABDOMEN
& DROPSY.

ASPHYXIA
Opium. *615*. *see CHEST*.

ASTHENOPIA
*SENSE OF WEAKNESS IN THE
EYES. see EYES*.

ASTHMA
SPASMODIC.

Ipec. *446*, Mag. phos. *525*. Nat.
sul. *582*.

VIOLENT.

Nat. sul. *581*.

NERVOUS.

Mag. phos. *525*.

HYSTERICAL.

Nux. mosch. *597*.

INFANTILE.

Vib. *866*.

IN CHILDREN.

Ars. (Nat. sul. *583*) Acon.
Cham, Ipec. Mosch, Puls.
Samb. Nat. sul. *584*.

IN CHILDREN OF SYCOTIC
PARENTS.

Nat. sul. *582*.

WITH TUBERCULOUS FAMILY
HISTORY.

Dros. *360*.

ATTACKS DURING SLEEP,
WITHOUT WAKING.

Sul. Lach. *496*.

LIES ON BACK, ARMS WIDE APART, TO RELIEVE BREATHING.
Psor. *673*.

LIES ON FACE TO RELIEVE.
Med. *532*.

ALTERNATING WITH SKIN ERUPTIONS.
Sul. *791*.

WITH:

yellow expectoration. Kali sul. *477*.

discharge of urine. Kreos *480*.

painful respiration. Ars. *93*.

difficult slow breathing. Ferr. *372*.

suffocation. Ipec. *437, 439*.

feeling chest would sink in. Ptelea. *680*.

feeling he will die. Psor *677*.

constrictive sensation in chest. Ars. *93*. Chel. *251*.

oppression of chest. Ars. *93*. Chel. *251*.

internal burning, externals cold. Carbo v. *211*.

stitches beneath right ribs. Chel. *251*.

spasms of diaphragm. Staph. *770*.

'pulsatilla' symptoms. Puls. *682*.

RESULT OF:

fit of anger. Cham. *241*.

earlier illness e.g. whooping cough. Carbo v. *209*.

sailors going on shore. *Brom. 138, 142* (see Kali br. *463*).

suppression of eczema. Ars. *97*.

vaccinations. Thuja. *826/7*.

WHERE ARSENICUM ONLY PALLIATES.
Nat. sul. Thuja. *820*.

CRAVES SALT.
Nat. mur (Ferr. phos *376*).
Nat. mur *571*.

UNABLE TO SPEAK OR SWALLOW.
Cup. *346*.

CHLOROSIS.
Calc. p. *167*.

CANNOT INSPIRE.
Iod. Brom. *138*.

CANNOT EXHALE.
Chlorum. Brom. *138*.

COUGH WITH HOARSENESS.
Ammon. carb. *42*.

AS IF HE WOULD DIE FOR WANT OF BREATH.
Ammon. carb. *46*.

FROM FATTY DEGENERATION OF HEART.
Arnica *89*.

> SITTING UP.
Kali carb. *470*.

> LEANING FORWARD.
Kali carb. *470. 473*.

< IN WARM ROOM.
Ammon carb. *46*.

> WALKING.
Ferr. *372*, Nux. v. *604*.

< GOING UP HILL.
Nux. v. *604*.

< AT SEASHORE.
Med. Brom. *138*. Nat. mur.
568.

> TALKING.
Ferr. *372*.

> CONSTANT READING AND
WRITING.
Ferr. *372*.

< DRY COLD WEATHER.
Hepar *403*.

> DAMP WEATHER.
Hepar 403.

< DAMP.
Nat. sul. (Hepar *403*) Nat. sul.
581.

< 3. A.M.
Kali carb. *470, 473*.

> STANDING BY OPEN WINDOW.
Ipec *444*.

ATELACTASIS
COLLAPSE OF PART OF THE
LUNG.
Ant. tart. *68*.

AVERSIONS
ACID FOOD.
Kreos. *480*.

ALCOHOL.
Con. *322. Ran. b. 702*.

BEER.
Alum. *35*. Asaf. *103*, Cycl. *351*,
Ferr. *372*. Sepia *741*. Kali bich.
455. Mez. *552/3*.

BREAD.
Con. *328*. Cycl. *250/1*, Lil. tig.
509, Nat. mur. *572*. nitric. ac.
591. Nat. sul. *584*. Nat. mur.
San. *734*. Sepia *741*.

BUTTER.
Cycl. *350/1*, Ptelea. *679*, Puls.
684.

CABBAGE.
Pet. *629*.

CAKE.
Ferr. phos. *386*.

CHEESE.
Ptelea. *680*.

COFFEE.
Aeth. *17*, Calc. *154*. Ferr. phos.
380. Ign. *425*. Lil. tig. *509*. Lyc.
515, Nat. mur. *572*. Nux. v. *605*.

EATING.
Ammon. carb. *43*.

EGGS.
Ferr. *372*.

EGGS COOKED IN ALUMINIUM
PANS.
Alum. *33*.

FISH.
Graph. *399*.

FOOD IN GENERAL.
Ant. tart. *65*. Ars. *99*. Alum. *37*.
Tub. *837*. Nux. v. *605*. Sang.
731. Sepia. *741*.

FOOD, OTHER THAN A VERY
LITTLE.
Cycl. *350/1*.

FOOD, DURING
CONVALESCENCE.
Kreos *480*.

FOOD — COOKED.
Graph. *399*.

FOOD — ANIMAL.
Graph *399*, Ptelea *679*.

HERRING.
Ferr., phos. *380*.

MEAT.

Tarent *801*, Alum. *35*. Calc. *154, 161*. Ferr. *372*. Ferr. phos. *380*. Kali bich. *459*, Lyc. *515*. Mur. ac. *563*. Nux. v. *609*. Pet. *629*, Ptelea. *680*. Sepia *741*.

MILK.

Aeth. *19*. Ant. tart. *65*. Calc. *154*, Ferr. *372*. Iris *451*. Nat. sul. *582*. Sepia *741*. Sil. *759*.

ONIONS.

(in sore throat) Alum. *35*. *Thuja. 826*. Thuja. (Lyc *521*).

OYSTERS.

Lyc. *515. 521*.

PASTRY AND RICH THINGS.

Puls. *686*.

PORK.

Cycl. *350*. Psor. *677*, Puls *685*.

PORK — FOR ILL EFFECTS OF EATING . . .

Puls *681*.

POTATOES.

Alum. Nat. sul. *582*. Alum. *36/7*. Loathing for. Alum. *39*.

RICE PUDDINGS.

Ptelea. *679. 680*.

SALT, VINEGAR, PEPPER.

Alum. *35*.

STARCHY FOOD.

Nat. sul. *582*.

STRAWBERRIES.

Oxal. acid (Lyc. *521*) (eat cheese to overcome ill effects of strawberries, tomatoes or oysters. Lyc. *521*).

SWEET THINGS.

Ver. vir. *858*, Graph. *399*, Ign. *425*.

VINEGAR, SOUR WINE OR FRUIT.

Ant. tart. *65*.

FATS.

Sepia. Nat. mur *570*. Phos. *641*, Sepia (Nitric ac. *586*). Pet *629*. Ptelea. *679*, Puls. *686*, Sepia *741*.

TOBACCO.

Nux. v. *605*. Calc. *154*. Ign. *425*.

TOBACCO SMOKE.

Alum. *35*. Ign. *430*.

DUST.

Lyssin (Hydrophobinum) Brom. *138*.

DRAUGHTS.

Brom. *138*.

READING.

Brom. *140*.

TO HAVING HEAD UNCOVERED.

PSor *678*.

TO OPEN AIR.

Calc. *163*, Coffea. *300*. Pet. *629*.

MENTAL EXERTION.

Bapt. *115*. Tub. *836*.

work.

Brom. *140*, Calc. *156*.

TO USUAL CIGAR.

Lil. tig. *509*.

TURPENTINE.

Tereb. *813*.

B

BACKACHE
(WHEN NOT FROM MECHANICAL CAUSES), SEE ALSO SPINE.

PAIN:
in and beneath right scapula. Chel. *251*.

in right shoulder. Chel. *251*.

with throbbing in abdominal and pelvic cavities. Aesc. *15*.

Shooting. Aesc. *15*.

Cutting. Aesc. *15*.

drawing. Cham. *241*.

dull. Aesc. *12*.

in sacroileac region. Aesc. *12*, Cham. *241*.

< stooping. Aesc. *12, 14*.

< in lower back. Aesc. *14*.

< walking, or any movement. Aesc. *14*.

> after continued movement. Rhus. Aesc. *15*.

< sitting. Agar. *22*.

< rising from sitting. Aesc. *12*.

LAMENESS AS IF STRAINED.
Aesc. *15*.

BAZIN'S
BLUE MARKS ON CALVES WITH ULCERS.
Dros *359*.

BESDORES
Bapt. *115*.

BLADDER
PAIN:
violent. Canth. *193. 198*.

burning. Caps. *199, 201*. Tereb *810. 811*.

< at rest, > walking in open air. Tereb. *811*.

short crampy intermittent. Caul *217*.

BURNING IN URETHRA DURING MICTURITION.
Ars. *99*.

TENESMUS
Caps. *201*. Pyrogen *691*.

STRANGURY
Canth. *193/4, 198*. Caps. *201*. Tereb. *813*.

PARALYSIS
Caust. *223*, Con. *322*.

HAEMORRHAGE FROM . . .
Ferr. phos. *380*.

CATARRH OF . . .
Dulc. *364*.

POLYPI AND VARICES OF . . .
Calc. *161*.

INVOLUNTARY MICTURITION.
Ars. *99*.

SCANTY EMISSION.
Ars. *99*.

WEAK, NO EXPULSIVE POWER.
Con. *322*, Opium. *616*.

CONSTANT DESIRE TO URINATE.
Lil. tig. *512*.

RENAL COLIC.
Lyc. *518*.

RENAL CALCULI.
Tereb. *812*.

IRRITATION OF LINING
    MEMBRANE OF . . .
    Plumbum 667.

FEELS FULL, AS IF CONTENTS
    WOULD FALL OUT.
    Sepia 743.

BLENORRHEA
EXCESSIVE DISCHARGE OF
    MUCUS. SEE LUNGS.

BLEPHARITIS
(INFLAMMATION OF EYELIDS)
    Staph. 762, Graph. 397 see
    EYES.

BLISTERS
ON FINGER TIPS.
    Ail 28.

PREVENTED WITH ONIONS.
    Allium 32.

BLOATING
OF WHOLE BODY.
    Aeth. 20. see ABDOMEN.

BLOOD POISONING
    Pyrogen 694. Anthracinum.
    (Pyrogen 697)

BLUSHING
    Ferr. 374.

BOILS
CROPS OF . . .
    Anthracinum. Tarent cub.
    Arn. Bellis, Sul. 782.

SUCCESSION OF . . .
    Nat. phos. 576 Sil. 751.

MANY SMALL BOILS.
    Arn. 91. Bellis 127. Abrot. 2.

WITH BURNING PAINS.
    Anthracinum. (Crot. 334)

WITH OEDEMA AROUND . . .
    Crot. 338.

WITH BLACK NON-COAGULABLE
    BLOOD.
    Crot. 338.

WITH BLUISH COLOUR AND
    INTENSE BURNING.
    Tarent. 805.

IN EXTERNAL EAR.
    Picric ac. 656.

THAT DO NOT MATURE.
    San. 735.

AS RESULT OF VACCINATIONS.
    Sil. 751. Thuja 826.

< HEAT OF BED.
    Merc. Sul. 782.

BONES
PAINS:
    Aur. 108/9, Dros. *358*, Ipec. *446*.

    in long bones. Dros. (Caust
    223) Dros. *358* Mez. *552*. Lach.
    Asaf. Mez. *555*.

    wander from bone to bone.
    Kali bich. *455*.

    in shinbones. (Syphilitic
    periostitis) Kali bich. *461*.

    syphilitic bone pains. Nitric
    ac. *593*.

    'growing pains' in . . . Phos.
    ac. *636, 639*.

    periostitis. Symphitum. *797*.
    rheumatic periostitis. Mez.

555, Asaf. Dros. Lach. Phyt.
652. Ruta. *722*.

as if broken. Theridion. *817*.

ACHING.
Ammon carb. *46*, Tub. *837*.

INFLAMED.
Mez. *552*, Phos. ac. *638*.

SWOLLEN.
Mez. *552*.

NECROSIS.
Phos. *643*

of jaw. Mez. *555*.

BRUISED.
Ruta. *719, 722*. Tub. *837*.

INJURIES TO PERIOSTEUM.
Ruta 719.

SPRAINS.
Ruta. *722*.

LESIONS AND FRACTURES.
Ruta *722*, Symphitum *794*.

BONES FEEL AS IF MADE OF
GLASS.
Thuja *829*.

BROKEN BONES THAT REFUSE
TO KNIT.
Calc. p. *170*, Symphitum. *793/
7*.

NON-UNION.
Calc. p. *167* Symphitum *793/7*.

FRACTURED.
Calc. p. *169, 170*. Symphitum
797.

DISEASE < AT NIGHT.
Merc. *538*, Mez. *552*.

CARIES.
Cistus *287*.

FEELING AS IF WALKING ON THE
ENDS OF HIS BONES.
Cham. *242*.

FEELING AS IF BONES WERE
SCRAPED WITH A KNIFE.
Phos ac. *639*.

WITHOUT STRENGTH.
Calc. *154*.

CURVATURE OF . . .
Calc. *156*, Symphitum *796*

softening of . . .
Calc. *156*.

IRREGULAR DEVELOPMENT
OF . . .
Calc. *156*.

DEFECTIVE NUTRITION OF . . .
Calc. p. *169*.

< DAMP WEATHER.
Mez. *552*.

< TOUCH.
Mez. *552*.

BOWELS
BURNING IN . . .
Ail *28* Caps. *199*.

INACTIVE.
Alum. *39*.

INFLAMMATION OF . . .
Canth. *195*.

INFLAMMATION OF . . . WITH
DIARRHOEIA.
Canth. *195*.

(TO RELAX THE BOWELS.)
Cean. *232*.

BRAIN

CEREBRO-SPINAL MENINGITIS.
Ail 27. Cicuta. Nat. sul. 582,
Ferr. phos 379. Cicuta 261, 265,
Ipec. 441.

MENINGITIS:
at start of . . . Ammon. carb.
44.

with body cold, cyanotic.
Ammon. carb. 44.

with weak pulse. Ammon.
carb. 44.

with sharp stinging pains.
Apis 73.

< heat. Apis 73.

after mechanical injuries.
Arnica. 88.

traumatic meningitis. Hyp
422.

basilar from suppressed ear
discharge. Stram. 772.

**PRESSIVE PAIN IN HALF OF
BRAIN AS FROM A PLUG OR
NAIL.**
Thuja. Hepar 405.

INFLAMMATION OF . . .
Canth. 195, Plumbum. 667.

STITCHING PAINS.
movement. Bry 144.

SOFTENING OF . . .
Phos 644, Plumbum. 669

FATTY DEGENERATION OF . . .
Picric ac. 655, Plumbum. 669.

FEELS LOOSE.
Hyos 415, Nat. sul. 584. Nux.
mosch. 597.

FEELS TIGHT.
Kali br. 467.

**FEELS CONSTRICTED AS BY A
LIGATURE.**
Cocc. 291.

CONCUSSION.
Arn. 90/1. Cicuta 261/2.

**DISTURBANCE RESULTING IN
PARALYSIS.**
Caust. 230.

TURMOIL IN TEMPER.
Cham. 236.

TURMOIL IN BRAIN.
Bell 116. (Cham. 236)

BRAIN FAG.
Ail 27. Picric ac. 656.

NUMB FEELING IN BRAIN.
Plat. 662.

**SENSATION OF FOREIGN BODY IN
SKULL.**
Con. 328, Iod. 433. > motion.
Iod. 433.

**SENSATION OF NAIL DRIVEN
INTO BRAIN.**
Thuja. 829. Thuja. Ptelea 679.

**SENSATION OF COLD CLOTH
ROUND BRAIN.**
San 733.

NUMB FEELING IN . . .
Plat. 662.

BREASTS
SEE FEMALE SEX.

BRIGHT'S DISEASE
Calc. Sul. 172.

BROMIDES
Kali br. *464.*

BRONCHITIS
Colch. *302.*

CHRONIC.
Ammon. carb. *44.*

DILATION OF BRONCHIAL
TUBES.
Ammon. carb. *44.*

OEDEMA.
Ammon carb. *44.*

OF SMALL CHILDREN.
Ant. tart. *59.*

CHEST FULL OF RATTLES AND
WHEEZES.
Ant. tart. *59.*

WITH VIOLENT SYMPTOMS.
Acon. Bell. Bry. Ant. tart. *64.*

WITH LITTLE FEVER, COLD
SWEAT.
Ant. tart. *64.*

BREATHING RATTLING,
ANXIOUS, WHEEZING.
Hepar *403.*

FETID BREATH.
Kreos *478.*

WITH EMPHYSEMA OF AGED.
Ledum. *502.*

BURNS
PAIN.
Canth. 196. Urtica Urens.
(Symphitum. *794*) Urtica *843.*

CICATRICES (SCARS)
ESPECIALLY OF BURNS.
Caust. *225.*

SUPERFICIAL.
Urtica *843.*

'NEVER BEEN WELL SINCE A
BURN'.
Caust *225.*

WITH BLISTERS.
Uritica. Canth. *196.*

TO PREVENT BLISTERS –
ONIONS.
Allium *32.*

BUTTERMILK
Calc. p. *169.*

C

CACHETIC CONSTITUTION
Calc. *163.*

CALCIUM
Ferr. phos. *376.*

CANCER
OF LIP.
Cistus *288.* Phyt. *652.*

OF CHEEK.
Con. *328.*

OF TONGUE.
Crot. *336.*

OF STOMACH.
Crot. *338.* Ornithogalum.
(Graph. *398*).

OF UTERUS.
Crot. *338.* Merc. *540.* Kreos
478. 482.

29

OF INTESTINES.
Graph. *397*.

OF HEART.
Kreos *482*.

OF MAMMAE.
Kreos *482*. Merc. *540*.

OF PYLORUS AND DUODENUM.
Ornithogalum. *619*. *620/1*.

OF CERVIX WITH VERY
OFFENSIVE ODOUR.
Kreos (Psor *675*).

SARCOMA OF FACE.
Symphitum. *795/6*.

PAINS OF.
Silica *757*.

SCIRRHUS.
Phyt *652*.

TUMOURS OF LIPS AND FACE.
Con. *328*.

SCIRRHUS PAINS, BURNING,
STINGING OR DARTING.
Apis. Con. *324*.

CANCEROUS TISSUE IRRITANT.
Alum. *35*.

ASSUAGING PAIN.
Ars. *95*.

WITH EMACIATION.
Brom. *140*.

THEORY OF ORIGIN OF . . .
Morb. *559*.

CANCRUM OVIS
See MOUTH.

CARDIALGIA
See HEART.

CARIES
See BONES.

CAROTIDS
THROBBING.
Bell *124*.

CARPHOLOGY
FITFUL PLUCKING MOVEMENTS
IN DELIRIUM
Hyos. *413*.

CATALEPSY
Cann. *179, 188/9, 192*. Ign. *425*.

CATAMENIA
(MENSTRUATION)
Borax *136*, Calc. *158, 161*. See
FEMALE SEX.

CATARACT
Ammon carb. *42*, Cina *284*.
Puls. Kali sul. *476*.

CATARRH
ACUTE.
Allium *30*.

CHRONIC.
Caps. *205*. Sil. Kali br. (Caps
205) Chel. *251*, Cistus *285*.

CHRONIC BRONCHIAL.
Hepar *407*.

CATARRHAL FEVER.
Hepar *406*.

VIOLENT.
Lyc, *517*.

ATROPHIC.
Mez. *556*.

SUFFOCATING.
Ant. crud. *55*. Ars. *93*. Lyc. *517*.

FREQUENT AND VIOLENT SNEEZING.
Cistus. *286*.

CATARRHAL DYSPNOEIA.
Ammon carb. *46*.

INFANTILE.
Calc. *160*.

GASTRIC.
Ant. crud. *53*. Chel. *251*, Ver. Alb. *854*.

FROM CHILLING STOMACH WITH ICE WATER WHEN HEATED.
Ars. Acon. *11*.

OF CHEST.
Agar. *21*, Ant. tart. *64*.

INTESTINAL.
Chel. *251*.

OF BLADDER.
Dulc. *364*.

NASAL.
Ign. *432*. Kali bich. *456*. Nitric ac. *590*. Tub. *834*.

WITH:
rough throat. Nux v. *604*.

headache. Nux v. *604*.

greenish discharges. Nat. sul. *581*.

yellow expectoration. Ammoniacum. Puls *686*. Ant. tart. *64*.

white expectoration. Ant. tart. *64*.

coryza. Bell *122*. Nux. v. *604*. Ran. b. *702*.

pressure in forehead above eyes. Cistus. *286*.

pain in joints. Ran. b. *702*.

< **COLD WET WEATHER.**
Dulc. *363/4 366*.

> **NOSE KEPT WARM.**
Dulc. *364*.

< **IN OPEN AIR.**
Dulc. *364*.

> **IN OPEN AIR.**
Puls *686*.

< **DURING EVENING.**
Allium *32*. Ars. *93*.

< **IN WARM ROOM.**
Allium *32*.

CELLULITIS
(**INFLAMMATION IN CELLULAR TISSUE**)
Canth. *197*, Arn. *87*.

CEREBRAL ANAEMIA
See ANAEMIA.

CHALYBEATE WATERS
HEALTH SPRINGS.
Ferr. *368*.

CHEST
PAIN:
on movement of trunk.

with heat. Ant. crud. *54*, Kreos. *481*. Med. *532*.

burning. Canth. *198*, > heat Ars. *94*, Kreos *480* Tereb. *810*.

cool. Camph. *176*.

stitching. Arn. *86*. Bry. *150*.

< pressure. Ran. b. *698/9*.

needle-like. Cham. *241*.

during INspiration. Calc. *162*, Kali carb. *473*. Ran. b. *699*.

in sternum. Cimic. *275*. Cina *283* Nat. phos *577* Phos ac. *638*.

in sternum. < walking Cimic *275*.

< for movement. Bry *144*. Bry. Ran. b. *698*.

> for pressure. Bry. Ran. b. *698*.

< in dry cold winds. Acon. Bry (Ran. b. *698*).

< wet weather. Ran. b. *698*.

< change of weather. Ran. b. *698*.

RHEUMATIC.
Ran. b. *699*.

BEHIND STERNUM WITH COUGH.
Sang. *730*.

THROUGH UPPER LEFT CHEST TO SHOULDER.
Sul. Pix liquida. Anisum stellatum Myrtis communis. Theridion. *818*.

IN A SPOT IN RIGHT CHEST.
Kali bich. *453*.

BURNING IN FIXED SPOT ON CHEST.
Ledum. *507*.

IN WHOLE OF RIGHT SIDE.
Chel. *251*.

WITH PAINFUL RESPIRATION.
Ars. *93*. Caps. *203*.

WITH DIFFICULT RESPIRATION.
Phos *646*. Psor *677*.

WITH SHORTNESS OF BREATH.
Kreos *480*. Phos *646*. Ant. tart. *67*.

DIFFICULTY IN BREATHING AFTER EXERCISE.
Arn. *86*. Ars. *93*, *99*.

SHORTNESS OF BREATH (See DYSPNOEIA).
Ars. *99*, Caust *228*. Ledum. *505*. Colch. *307*, Ipec. *445*.

UNEQUAL BREATHS.
Ant. tart. *67*.

SHORT QUICK BREATHING.
Chel. *251*.

> **DEEP INSPIRATIONS.**
Chel. *251*.

DOUBLE INSPIRATION.
Ledum. *507*.

OPPRESSIVE PAIN < **BREATHING.**
Dulc. *366*, Ferr *371/2*. Glon. *393*. Sepia *742*. Med. *532*.

SIGHING.
Camph. *176*.

SLOW AND IRREGULAR RESPIRATION.
Opium. *615*.

CHEYNE-STOKES RESPIRATION.
Opium. *614*.

CONTINUAL STERTORIUS RESPIRATION.
Opium. *614*.

SHORT OF BREATH.
< walking. Sul. *780*.

< in evening in bed. Sul. *780*.

wants doors and windows wide open. Sul. *780*.

BREATHING DIFFICULT, PAINFUL.
Bry. Ver. vir. *862*, Acon. *10*.

SLOW.
Cocc. *291*.

BURNING ALONG STERNUM.
Tereb. *810*.

CONGESTED.
Ferr. phos *379*. Sul. *780*, Agar. *22*, Ars. *93*. Asaf. *101*. *103*. Aur. *110*. Brom. *142*. Cocc. *297*. Colch. *305*. Caust *228*. Ferr. *371*, Camph. *176*. Caps. *201*, *202*. Graph. *400*, Ver. vir. *860*. with palpitations. Glon. *393*.

RECURRING TIGHTNESS OF CHEST.
Ars. *93*. Asaf. *102*. Caust *228*. Ran. b. *699*. Cham *241*.

VIOLENT PAIN ABOVE LEFT NIPPLE ON RISING.
Ran. b. *700*.

PAIN AS IF BRUISED IN REGION OF SHORT RIB.
Ran. b. *700*.

PRESSURE IN CHEST.
Phos *645*. *646*. Sul. *780*.

RATTLING OF MUCOUS.
Calc. *162*.

CHEST FILLS WITH MUCOUS.
Cistus. *287*.
when empty feels raw. Cistus *287*.

FULL OF MUCOUS.
Ant. tart. *64*, *67*.

FEELS HOLLOW.
Cocc. *298*.

FEELS TOO NARROW.
Nux. Mosch. *598*

COLDNESS, PROSTRATION, WEAKNESS.
Ammon carb. *46*.

ACUTE INFLAMMATION OF RESPIRATORY TRACT.
Ant. tart. *59*.

DIAPHRAGMITIS.
Cactus, Ran. b. *702*. Stram. *777*.

STITCHES AND INFLAMMATIONS.
Kali. carb. *470*.

CONSTRICTION AS FROM AN IRON BAND.
Cactus. (Gel *384*) Merc. *543*.

FEELING CHEST WOULD BURST.
San. *735*.

FEELING CHEST IS HOLLOW.
Sepia *743*.

FEELING LIKE A BIG EMPTY CASK.
Phyt. *652*.

FEELING OF BAND ROUND CHEST.
Aeth. *20*.

STITCHES BETWEEN RIBS.
Staph. *764*.

MUCOUS RALES IN BOTH LUNGS.
Phos *646*.

CONSTANT RALES.
Ant. tart. *61*. Phos *646*.

RATTLING PLUS COLD BREATH AND EXTREMITIES.
Carbo v. Ant. tart. *62*. *64*. *70*.

loud rattling with paralysis.
Moschus. Ant. tart. *62*. Ipec.
Ant. tart. *64*.

RATTLING OF PHLEGM.
Baryta carb. Ant. tart. *62, 67*,
Kali hyd. Ant. tart *62*. *64*.

BUBBLINGS IN CHEST.
Ant. tart. *63*.

DULL PRESSURE.
Phos ac. *638*. Anac. *48/9*.
Kreos *480*, Lyc. *519*.

SWOLLEN.
Bell *122*.

SORE.
Calc. 155, 162, Caust *228*.

WITH PALPITATION.
Colch. *307*.

ASPHYXIA FROM PARALYSIS OF
DIAPHRAGM AND
RESPIRATORY MUSCLES.
Con. *331*.

ORTHOPNEA.
Ant. tart. *62*.

ACCUMULATION OF FLUID IN
SEROUS MEMBRANES.
Apis. Bry. Sul. Ran. b. *700*.

PLEURODYNIA.
Arn. Colc. *303, 307*, Cimic *274*.
Arn. (Ran. b. *698*). Ran. b,
699.

HYDROTHORAX.
Colch. *308/9*.

EXPECTORATION.
yellowish green. Psor *677*.

THORAX SEIZED WITH
SPASMODIC CONTRACTIONS.
Asaf. *101*.

CHEST SYMPTOMS
ALTERNATING WITH FISTULO
IN ANO.
Calc. p. *166*.

WEAK FATIGUED FEELING.
Carbo v. *212*.
< waking. Carbo v. *212*.

SERIOUS EFFUSIONS IN CHEST.
Colch. *309*.

PULMONARY HAEMORRHAGE.
Collin. *310*.

INFLAMMATIONS OF CHEST.
Ars. *93*.

OPPRESSION OF . . .
Dros *361*.

OPPRESSION GOING UP HILL.
Ars. *94*.

TICKLING BEHIND STERNUM.
Con. *329*, San. *735*. Staph. *764*.

SORE NIPPLES.
Arn. *89*.

ONE NIPPLE SWOLLEN AND
PAINFUL.
Sil. *752*.

PULMONARY ABSCESS.
Hepar *407*.

EMPYEMA.
Hepar *407*.

PYOTHORAX.
Hepar *407*.

RATTLING IN BRONCHI.
Ipec. *445*.

RATTLING WITH COUGH.
Kali sul. *476*.

WITH INCLINATION TO VOMIT.
Ipec. *445*.

ULCERATION OF LUNGS.
Kali carb. *473.*

HYDROPERICARDIUM.
Ars. Lyc. *519.*

MUST SIT UP IN BED TO COUGH.
Phos. *646.*

CANNOT BEAR WEIGHT OF
ARMS ON CHEST.
Psor. *672.*

> LYING DOWN.
Psor. *677.*

SENSATION OF LUNGS ON
FIRE . . .
> fresh air. Pyrogen. *691.*

AILMENTS AFFECTING RIGHT
LUNG.
Sang. *730/1.*

EXTREME EXTERNAL
TENDERNESS.
Ran. sc. (Ran. b. *703*).

GNAWING IN LEFT SIDE OF . . .
Ruta *721.*

CATARRHAL IRRITATION IN . . .
Sang. *729.*

SENSATION OF HEAVY LOAD ON
CHEST.
Ver. vir. *862.*

OPPRESSION OVER WHOLE
CHEST.
Vib. *865.*

SORE SPOTS IN CHEST
FOLLOWING PNEUMONIA.
Ran. b. *702.*

CHILBLAINS
BURNING.
Sul *782.*

PAINFUL.
Agaricus *23*, Pet. *629, 633.*

ITCHING.
Nux, v., Agar. Abrot. *2.* Pet
629, 631, Ruta *717.* Agar. *25.*

BLUE.
Puls. (Kali sul. *476*).

PURPLE.
Pet *631.*

ON HEEL.
Pet *632.*

< COLD.
Agar. *23* (Kali sul *476*).

< WARM.
Puls *687* (Agar *23*) (Kali sul.
476).

CHILDREN
CANNOT BEAR TO BE TOUCHED
OR LOOKED AT.
Cina *281*, Cham *238.* Ant.
crud *52.* Ant. tart. *61/2. 64. 66.
69.*

EXTREMELY IRRITABLE.
Ant. tart. *64*, Cham. *238.*

"CAN'T BEAR . . . PEOPLE,
PAIN, ETC."
Cham. *236.*

DESIRES THINGS BUT REFUSES
THEM WHEN OFFERED.
Bry. Staph. Cina *281.*

CHILDREN WHO ARE SNAPPISH,
WITH EARACHE.
Cham. Allium *31.*

CHILDREN WHO CRY PITIFULLY
AND HAVE EARACHE.
Puls. (Allium. *31*).

CHILDREN WHO WANT TO BE
CARRIED.
Cham. Ant. tart. *62, 67.*
Cham. *238, 241.* Cina, *281, 283.*

PEEVISH.
Cham. *238.*

RESTLESS.
Cham. *238,* Cina *281.*

VERY SENSITIVE TO TOUCH.
Acon *11.* Ant. tart. *61.*

COUGH AS RESULT OF GETTING
ANGRY.
Ant. tart. *61.*

MARASMIC, YET WITH
VORACIOUS APPETITE.
Bar. carb. Sil. Nat. mur. Sul.
Calc. iod. Abrot. *1.*

DELICATE CHILDREN.
Alum. *39.*

UNABLE TO HOLD HEAD UP.
Abrot. Aeth. *18.*

BABIES WHO WILL NOT SLEEP
DAY OR NIGHT.
Psor. *672, 678.*

BABIES GOOD ALL DAY,
RESTLESS, TROUBLESOME,
SCREAMING ALL NIGHT.
Psor. *672. 678.*

CHILD WANTS TO NURSE ALL
THE TIME, YET LOSES FLESH.
Nat. mur. Abrot. San. *733.*

AFTER FEEDING, VOMITS, AND
THEN GOES TO SLEEP.
Aeth. Ipec. San. *734.* Aeth. *19.*

BABIES WHO CANNOT
TOLERATE MILK.
Aeth. *17. 19.*

CHILDREN WHO CRAVE BREAD
BOILED IN MILK.
Abrot. *1.*

INFANTS THAT ARE FED EVERY
TIME THEY CRY.
Aeth. cynapium. Aeth. *18.*

CONVULSIONS OF TEETHING
CHILDREN.
Acon. *11.*

CRY BEFORE URINATING.
San. *735.*

URINE STAINED RED.
Lyc. San. *735.*

CRAVES WATER.
San. 734.

POT-BELLIED.
San. *734.*

GROW TOO FAT.
Calc. carb. (Phos ac. *636*).

GROW TOO TALL AND FAST.
Phos. ac. *636.*

ROSY, CHUBBY, PLETHORIC
BABIES.
Acon. *6.*

'IDIOTIC' CHILDREN.
Aeth. *17.*

UNDER-NOURISHED, FACE
PINCHED AND OLD-LOOKING.
Sil. *755.*

PRECOCIOUS.
Bell *124.*

KICKS OFF CLOTHING IN
COLDEST WEATHER.
Sul. San. *735.*

HYDROCELE IN . . .
Rhod. Abrot. *2.*

36

BRONCHITIS AND BRONCHO-
PNEUMONIA.
Ant. tart. *59*.

CHLOASMA
BROWN BLOTCHES ON FACE,
CHIEFLY IN PREGNANT
WOMEN. See
PREGNANCY.

CHLOROSIS
FORM OF SIMPLE ANAEMIA.
Calc. *157. 164* Calc. p. *166. 169*.

CHOLERA
Camph. *174, 176/7*. Cup *343*.
SPASMODIC.
Cup. 344.
CONVULSIVE.
Cup. *344*.
WITH EXTREME COLDNESS.
Camphor (Cup. *344*).
WITH COPIOUS SWEAT.
Veratrum. (Cup. *344*). Ver.
alb. *854*.
IN EARLY STAGES.
Camphor. (Cup. *348*).
CHOLERA ASIATICA. SUL. *789*,
Carbo. v. *212*. Ver. alb. *854*.
EARLY STAGES WITH
COLLAPSE, COLDNESS &
SUDDEN PROSTRATION.
Camphor (Ver. alb *857*).
WITH EXCESSIVE CRAMPS.
Cuprum. (Ver. alb. *857*).
WITH EXCESSIVE COLD.
Ver. alb. *857*.

RESULT OF USING COPPER
UTENSILS.
(Cup *344*).
CHOLERA INFANTUM, WITH
GREEN WATERY STOOLS.
Aeth. *15*. Calc. *160*. Calc. p.
166. Sal. ac. *725*.
CHOLERA INFANTUM (ENTERO-
COLITIS).
Iris. *450*. kali br. *467*. Nux
Mosch. *599*. Opium. *616*.
Phyt. *652*. Kreos. *482. 484*.
Med. *531*.

CHOREA
(ST VITUS' DANCE)
Cimic. *270*, Caul. *219*. Stram.
769. Hyos. *408. 415*. Agar. *21/2
25*. Ign. *426*.
TWITCHING OF MUSCLES.
Hyos. Stram. Mygale. Ign.
Agar. *23*.
CONSTANT STATE OF ERETHISM.
Hyos. *408*.
JERKINGS.
Hyos. *408*.
WITH GYRATORY MOVEMENTS.
Stram. (Hyos. *408*).
WITH SPASMS.
Hyos. *415*. Mag. phos. *524*.
DROPS THINGS.
Agar. *22*.
WITH:
headaches. Agar. *24*.
trembling spells. Calc. *158*.
irregular menses. Cimic. *272*.
paralytic weakness. Cocc. *294*.

convulsive paroxysms. Tereb.
811.

OF LEFT LEG, ARM, FACE.
< at approach of a storm.
Rhod. *705*.

IN CHRONIC DISEASES.
Sul. *791*.

OF BODY.
Ver. vir. *862*. Vib. *867*.

OF THE HEART.
Tarent. *808*.

OF BODY, UNAFFECTED BY
SLEEP.
Ver. vir. *862*.

OF BODY, BUT NO MOTION OF
EYES WHEN ASLEEP.
Agar. *25*.

CHOROIDITIS.
INFLAMMATION OF CHOROID
COAT OF THE EYE, AND
POSSIBLY OF THE IRIS. See
EYES.

CHRONIC ACID
Kali bich. *455/6*.

CHRONIC DISEASES
THEORY
Morb. *558*. *560*. Tub. *840*.

CICATRICES
SCARS.
Caust. *225*.

CINCHONA BARK
China. *253*. *256*.

CLAIRVOYANCE
Cann. *191*.

COD LIVER OIL
Calc. p. *170*.

COLD
< FROM COLD.
Bell. *117*. *119*. Brom. *140*. *142*.
Caps. *205*. Cistus. *286*. Caul.
219. Psor. *674*. Pyrogen *691*.
Cimic. *276*.

> FROM COLD.
Iodum. (Brom. *138*) Ledum.
501. Glon. (Bell. *117*).

ALWAYS CHILLY.
Cimic. *276*, Kali carb. *469*.
472. Sil. *751*. *755*.

CREEPING CHILLINESS, BEFORE
A COLD.
Merc. *538*.

CHILLS FROM EVERY
MOVEMENT.
Nux. v. (Merc. *538*).

CHILL, WITH REDNESS OF FACE.
Ign. *431*.

COLD LIMBS.
Carbo v. *211*. Cham. *242*.
Pyrogen. *691*.

COLDNESS, WITHOUT
EXTERNAL CHILLINESS.
Ledum. *501*.

COLD IN SPOTS.
Pet. *631*.

VERY SENSITIVE TO COLD.
Psor. *678*.

CHILL BETWEEN SCAPULAE
BECOMES GENERAL
COLDNESS OF BONES AND
EXTREMITIES.
Pyrogen. *695*.

SCALP COLD.
has to wear a hat. Psor. *674*.

COLD, < AT NOON.
Kali carb. *468*.

COLD IN PATCHES.
Calc. *154*.

AFTER EVERY DRINK.
Caps. *203*.

< FROM BATHING.
Caps. *204*.

EXTERNALLY, WITH FEELINGS
OF INTERNAL HEAT.
Carbo. v. *211*.

INTERNAL HEAT, WITH
SHIVERING.
Cham. *242*.

FEELING OF BURNING ON
EXTERNAL COLD PARTS.
Secale (Ledum. *501*).

WITH HOT HEAD.
Arnica. (Ledum. *503*).

WITH HOT FACE AND BREATH.
Cham. *242*.

SENSATION OF COLDNESS IN
ULCERS.
Sil. (Merc. *538*).

COLDS

ALWAYS CATCHING COLDS.
Cistus *285* (repeat
periodically) Phos. ac. *635*.
Silica. *754*. Tub. *835*. China
260.

FROM EXPOSURE TO COLD AIR.
Kali carb. *468*.

< COLD AIR.
Cistus *285*. Phos. Rumex
(Cistus *286*).

EARLY COLDS.
Allium *30*. Ferr. phos *377*.

SUDDEN CHILLS.
Camphor *173*. Acon. (Gels
384).

AFTER DAMP COLD WINDS.
Allium *30*.

SOME HOURS AFTER EXPOSURE.
Gels. *384*.

FREQUENT AND VIOLENT
SNEEZING.
Cistus *285*. Allium. *30*.

SETTLE ON CHEST.
Phos. ac. *635*.

ALWAYS SETTLE IN THROAT.
Cistus *288*.

WITH:
vomiting. Cocc. *296*.
constant nasal drip. Euph.
(Allium *30*).
bland discharge from eyes.
Euph. (Allium *30*).
acrid discharge from eyes.
Allium *30*.
discharge that makes upper
lip raw. Allium *30*.
headache. Allium *30*.

< EVENINGS.
Allium *30*.

< INDOORS.
Allium *30*.

> OUT OF DOORS.
Allium *30*.

**HAYFEVER — MORNING COUGH
WITH VIOLENT SNEEZING IN
AUGUST.**
Allium *30*.

CHILLS:
as result of . . . Acon *5. 8*.

of whole body, with hot
forehead. Acon. *11*.

violent, with dry heat. Acon.
11.

COLIC
PAINS:
cutting. Ver. alb. *854*.

an hour or two after eating.
Nux. v. *608*.

neuralgic. Coloc. *314*.

as if sharp stones were
rubbing against each other in
abdomen. Cocc. *298*. Coloc.
313.

in hypogastrium. Acon. *12*.
Collin. *313*.

burning. Acon. *12*. Ver. alb.
854.

griping, cutting pains
> bending double. Kali carb.
471. Coloc. Caust *225*.

> at night. Coloc. Caust. *225*.

paroxysmal. Coloc. *315*.

tearing and cutting. >
evacuation. Dulc. *365*.

very violent. Opium *616*.

FROM:
taking cold. Dulc. *365*.

cold wet weather. Dulc. *365*.

eating acid fruit. Cistus. *285*.

eating ices. Calc. p. *168*.

FLATULENCE.
Acon. *12*. Aesc. *14*. Agar. *22*.
Cocc. *293. 296*. Ipec. *445*. Mag.
phos. *525*. Nat. sul. *585*. Puls.
684.

< EATING.
Colch. *302, 309*. Coloc. *314*.

WITH:
belching. Mag. phos. *525*.

constipation. Opium. *616*.

Convulsions. Cicuta. *262*.

diarrhoeia. Coloc. *314*.

fainting. Collin. *313*.

paralysis of lower extremities.
Plumbum. *664*.

urging to stool. Staph. *763*.

vomiting. Cicuta *262*. Coloc.
314/5.

PERIODIC.
Cham. *240*.

WIND OR MENSTRUAL COLIC.
Cocc. *293*, Mag. phos. *525*.
Coloc. *318*.

OF CHILDREN.
Nat. phos *576*.

**OF INFANTS. > LYING ON
STOMACH.**
Coloc. *316*.

**OF BABIES WITH CUTTING
TEARING PAINS.**
Allium *31*.

RESULT OF ANGER.
Cham. *Coloc 314/5*.

RESULT OF INDIGNATION.
Staph. *763*.

AFTER LITHOTOMY.
Staph. *763*.

PAINTER'S COLIC.
Plat.   *662*.

NEAR UMBILICUS.
Ipec. *445*. Nat. sul. *585*.

EVERY NIGHT. Iris *449*.

> HEAT.
Cham. *241*. Mag. phos. *527*.

> BENDING OVER.
Coloc. 314.

> PRESSING ABDOMEN.
Coloc *314*, Mag. phos *527*.

NO BETTER PRESSING
ABDOMEN.
Cham. (Coloc. *314*).

> MOTION.
Coloc *314*.

> FLATUS.
Coloc *318*.

> DURING REST, SITTING OR
LYING.
Nux. v. *605*.

> BENDING BACKWARDS.
Diosc. Plumbum. *665*.

< FOOD AND DRINK.
Staph. *763*.

COLITIS
MEMBRANOUS.
Colch. *303*.

ULCERATIVE.
Lil. tig. *511*.

ENTERO-COLITIS.
Tereb. *810*.

with haemorrhages and
ulceration of bowels. Tereb.
810.

CONCUSSION
Arn. *90*, Cicuta *262*. *264/6*.

WITH SPASMS.
Cicuta *266*.

CONDYLOMATA
SWELLINGS OF MUCOUS
MEMBRANES, See
MUCOUS
MEMBRANES.

CONGESTION OF BRAIN
Ail *27*. Bell *124*. Cimic. *273*.

WITH THREATENED
CONVULSIONS.
Apis *73*.

< BATHING IN HOT WATER.
Apis *73*

SPINAL.
Ail *27*.

CONSTIPATION
CHRONIC.
Opium. *616*.

TERRIBLE PAIN FROM
CONSTRICTION.
Plumbum *668*.

OBSTINATE.
Bry. *149*, Collin. *313*, Nat.
mur. *573*.

NO DESIRE FOR STOOL.
Alumina *35*, Bry. (Nux v.
606).

41

**NO POWER TO STRAIN FOR
STOOL.**
Alumina *35*.

**FREQUENT TENESMUS WITHOUT
BEING ABLE TO EXPEL
ANYTHING.**
Anac. *49*.

**NOT NORMALLY
CONSTIPATED.**
Puls. *686*.

WITH:
hard dry knotty white stools.
Aesc. *14*. Bry. *145*, Graph. *395*.
Ver. alb. *854*.

haemorrhoids. Collin. *311*,
3123, Aesc. (Collin *313*).

flatulence. Collin. *313*. Nat.
mur. *573*.

craving for salt and fat. Nitric
ac. *586*.

colic. Plumbum. *666*.

sensation of lump in rectum.
Sepia *747*.

**ALTERNATING WITH
DIARRHOEIA.**
Ant. crud. *53*, Cimic *273*, Tub.
837.

FROM:
irregular peristaltic action of
intestines. Nux. v. *606*.

lack of peristaltic action of
intestines. Opium. *615*.

lack of secretions in intestines.
Bry. (Nux. v. *606*).

constriction of intestines.
Nux. v. *606*.

OF SUCKLINGS.
Alum. *36*.

OF PAINTERS.
Plumbum. *666*

WHILE TRAVELLING.
Plat. *661*.

AFTER LEAD POISONING.
Plat. *661*.

DURING GESTATION.
Collin. *310*.

CONSTRICTION
OF THROAT. < LIQUIDS.
Bell. *124*.

OF ANUS.
Bell. *124*.

OF OS UTERI.
Bell. *124*.

CONSUMPTION
Med. *531*, Tub *831*, *836*.

CONVULSIONS
Abrot. *1*. (see also
EPILEPSY) Arn. *90*, Hyos
414.

OF TEETHING CHILDREN.
Acon. *11*.

OF INFANTS.
Bell *119*, *124*.

OF FISTS AND LEGS.
Glon. *390*.

OF FACIAL MUSCLES.
Cicuta *262*.

OF EXTENSOR MUSCLES.
Cina. *283*.

FROM FINGERS TO HANDS TO REST OF BODY.
Cicuta *265*.

STARTING IN FINGERS AND THUMBS.
Cup. *343*.

WHERE LIMB FIRST FLEXES AND THEN CONTRACTS.
Cup *345*.

AFTER LOSS OF SLEEP.
Cocc. *294. 297.*

AFTER PAIN IN REGION OF WOMB.
Collin. *311.*

WITH:

stiffness of limbs. Mag. phos *525.*

thumbs drawn in. Mag. phos *525.*

fingers clenched. Mag. phos. *525.*

paralysis. Plumbum. *669.*

mania. Ver. vir. *861.*

opisthotonos Nux. v. *607*, Phyt. *652*. Tereb. *811*. Ver. vir. *860*. Aeth. *20*. Arg. nit. *81,* Bell. *124,* Camph. *176, Cicuta 261/3 269*. Ign. *425*. Ipec. *441.*

left fingers spread apart. Glon. *390.*

AS RESULT OF VERMIFUGES.
Cina. *280.*

AS RESULT OF FRIGHT.
Ign. *426.*

AS RESULT OF SHOCK TO PIT OF STOMACH.
Cicuta *263.*

FROM NERVOUS EXCITEMENT.
Cimic *276.*

SUDDEN, AFTER SUPPRESSED DISCHARGES.
Cup. *345.*

AFTER SLIGHTEST TOUCH.
Nux. v. *607.*

FRIGHTFUL.
Stram. *775.*

VIOLENT, WITH HORRIBLE DISTORTIONS OF THE FACE.
Stram. *778.*

EXCESSIVELY VIOLENT.
Cicuta *261*. Bell. *116*. Cicuta *266.*

PUERPERAL.
Cham. *240,* Glon. *393*. Ver. vir. *861.*

IN WEAK SUBJECTS.
Calc. p. *169.*

ECLAMPSIA.
Calc. *156. 160*. Cicuta. *261.*

EXTENDS FROM CENTRE TO CIRCUMFERENCE. CICUTA *265.*

EXTENDS FROM ABOVE, DOWNWARDS.
Cicuta *265.*

EXTENDS FROM BELOW UPWARDS.
Cup. (Cicuta *265*).

SPASM FOLLOWED BY PATIENT APPEARING TO BE DEAD.
Cup. *343.*

BETWEEN CONVULSIONS:
mild, placid, Cicuta *265.*
irritable. Nux. v. Strych. (Cicuta *265*).

TONIC AND CLONIC.
Cocc. *291*.

> COOL ROOM.
Glon. *394*. Opium. *613*.

NEEDS TO BE UNCOVERED.
Opium. *613*.

ALTERNATING WITH RAGE.
Stram. *775*.

< HEAT.
Opium. Apis *73*. Opium. *614*.

CORDEE
INFLAMMATORY PAINFUL
DOWNWARD CURVING OF
PENIS.
Caps *201*.

CORNS
Ammon. carb. *42*.

CORPSE REVIVER
Carbo v. *206*.

CORYZA
THIN, WATERY, BURNING.
Ars. Aesc. *15*. Allium. *30*.

RAW.
Aesc. *15*. Allium. *30*.

STINGING AND BURNING.
Aesc. *15*.

EXCORIATING.
Cepa. Allium *30*.

ACRID LACHRYMATION.
Euphrasia, Allium *30*. Lac.
can. *488*.

DRY, STUFFED.
Ammon. carb. *44*. Sepia *740*.

FLUENT.
Bry *149*. Caust. *226*. Dulc. *363*.
Iod. *433*. Nux. v. *604*. Mez.
553.

DRY, WITH STOPPAGE OF·NOSE.
Caust. *226*. Dulc. *363*.

WITH:
congestion. Allium *30*.

pain in jaw and face. Allium.
30.

frontal and occipital
headaches. Allium *30*.

tears from eyes. Allium *30*.

cough. Bry *149*.

bland discharge. Euphrasia.
Allium *30*.

copious lachrymation.
Euphrasia. Allium *30*.

sneezing. Allium *30*. Nux. v.
604. Puls. *684*. Rhus *712*.

thick yellow mucous. Cistus
287. Theridion. *816*.

DURING DAY BUT NOT AT
NIGHT.
Nux. v. *604*.

IN MORNING.
Nux. v. *604*. Rhus. *712*.

AFTER BLOWING NOSE IT
BECOMES RAW.
Cistus *287*.

> FILLING UP WITH MUCOUS
AGAIN.
Cistus. *287*.

HAS TO BREATHE WITH MOUTH
OPEN.
Amon carb. *44*.

LONG CONTINUED.
Brom. *141*.

COUGHS

HOARSE.
Acon *10*, Bell. *122*. Caps. *201*.
Caust. *242*. Cina *283*, Kali
bich. *458*.
< morning. Caust. *222*.
< evening. Phos. (Caust *222*).

CONVULSIVE.
Agar. *21/2*. Iod *434*.

VIOLENT.
Agar. *21*, Borax *137*, Dros. *355*.
Kali bich. *460*.

CONTINUAL DRY.
Alum. *36*. Ammon. carb. *44*.
Bry *149*, Hyos. *414*, Cimic.
272.

HACKING.
Alum. *36*. Bry. *149*. Pet *631*.

DRY.
Ammon. carb. *43*, Bry. *145*.
Iod. *433*. Pet. *631*. Phos. *642*.
Phos. ac. *638*.

LOOSE.
Ant. tart. *61*. Nat. sul. *583*.

RATTLING.
Ant. tart. *64. 66*.

SPASMODIC.
Ipec. *443*. Mag. phos. *525*.
Mez. *553*. Caps. *201, 203*.
Chel. *249*. Dros. *355*. Hyos.
411. Kreos. *480*. Sepia *742*.
Bry. *145*. Cina *280*. Ferr. *371*.

SPASMODIC < SWALLOW OF
COLD WATER.
Caust *224. 228*.

SCRATCHY.
Cann. *183*.

PAROXYSMAL, VIOLENT.
Dros. *362*, Hepar *405, 407* Kali
carb. *470*. Caps. *205*. Carbo v.
211, Con. *327*, Kali bich. *460*.

TICKLING.
Sang. *729*. Calc. *157*.

ASTHMATIC.
Ipec. *443*, Kali carb. *473*.

STICKING IN CHEST AFTER
COUGHING.
Borax. *137*.

DRY, WITH SNEEZING.
Cina *282*.

DRY, HACKING.
Nitric ac. *592*, Phos. *645*. Sepia
742, Sang. *729*.

HOLLOW.
Bell. *122*.

TEARING COUGH LIKE
WHOOPING COUGH.
Ipec. Castenea. Tarent. *807*.

DEEP, EXHAUSTING.
Ail. *28*, Dros. *355*.

COUGH OF FLU.
Ammon. carb. *41*.

FIRST ATTACK SEVERE,
SUBSEQUENT ONES WEAKER.
Ant. crud. *54*.

WHEN HUNGRY.
Ant. tart. *65*.

COMPELLED TO SIT UP TO
COUGH.
Ant. tart. *66/7*.

NERVOUS COUGHS.
Caps. *201*.

FOLLOWING LOSS OF
CONSCIOUSNESS.
Cup. *346*.

THREATENING TO SUFFOCATE.
Cup. *346*.

1ST. COUGH SEVERE,
FOLLOWING ONES WEAKER.
Ant. crud. *54*.

WITH:

involuntary urination. Caust. *224*.

stitches in affected parts. Caps. *205*.

constriction in chest. Agar. *21*, Phos. *645*.

inability to expectorate. Con. *329*. Caust. *222*.

expectoration of blood. Kreos. *480*.

expectoration of green mucous. Psor. *676*.

expectoration lumpy yellow, green. Sil. *750*.

expectoration stringy. Kali bich. *458*.

dry throat. Sang. *729*.

sweats. Agar. *21*, Hepar *403*, Kali bich. *460*.

vomiting. Alum. *36*. Cina *280*. Dros. *355*.

arrest of breathing. Alum. *36*.

stitches in small of back. Ammon. carb. *42*.

burning in chest. Ammon. carb. *42*.

blood streaked sputa. Ant. tart. *68*, Ferr. *372*. Iod. *441*.

nosebleed. Ferr. phos. *380*.

dyspnoea. Kali bich. *458*.

itching behind sternum. Kali bich. *460*.

great pain in left chest. Nat. sul. *583*.

great pain in right chest. Kali sul. (Nat. sul. *583*).

clear blood. Ferr. phos. *380*.

pain through to back. Kali bich. *458*.

pain in some distant part. Caps. *200, 202/3*.

bursting headache. Caps. *201, 203*.

offensive breath. Caps. *201. 203*.

urine spurting during cough. Caust. *222*, Kreos. *480*, Colch. *309*.

tumour on neck. Cistus *285*.

FROM:

getting wet. Dulc. *363*.

cold damp weather. Dulc. *363*.

pressure on larynx. Lach. *498*.

tickling in throat. Ammon. carb. *42*, Iod. *433*. Ipec. *445*. Lyc. *519*.

inhaling cold air. Cup. *345*.

eating oysters. Lyc. *521*.

tightness of chest, suffocative. Hepar *406*. Iod. *434*, Ipec. *438*.

'TEETHING' COUGHS.
Calc. *153*.

CHILD CALLS OUT AFTER
COUGHING.
Cina. *283*.

IN CHILDREN.
Cup. *346*.

CHILD BECOMES RIGID AND
TURNS BLUE.
Ipec. *443*.

SPRINGS UP IN BED WITH
COUGH.
Bry. Nat. sul. *583*.

LIES ON FACE TO RELIEVE.
Med. *531*.

SENSATION AS IF HEAD IN A
BLANKET.
Sang. *730*.

WAKES HIM UP AT NIGHT.
> if he sits up and passes
flatus. Sang. *731*.

WHENEVER BODY IS
UNCOVERED.
Hepar. *407*.

CAUSING PAIN IN EPIGASTRIUM.
Nux. v. *604*.

AS IF CHEST WOULD FLY TO
PIECES WHEN COUGHING
DEEPLY.
Sul. *784*.

CAUSED BY LOUD SPEAKING.
Cocc. *298*.

CAUSED BY READING ALOUD.
Phos. *645*.

CAUSED BY BRUSHING TEETH.
Cocc. *298*.

FOLLOWING FEELINGS OF
APPREHENSION AND
DISCOURAGEMENT.
Rhus. *712*.

NOCTURNAL, DRY COUGH.
Puls. *685*.

ENDING IN VIOLENT SNEEZING.
Agar. *21*.

AFTER FLU.
Bry. Alum carb. *41*.

FEELS ABDOMEN WILL BURST.
Anac. *49*.

SLEEPINESS AFTER . . .
Anac. *49*.

APPARENT WEAKNESS OF
LUNGS.
Ant. tart. *64*.

< PUTTING HAND OR FOOT OUT
OF BED.
Hepar. *404*.

< COUGHING, WHICH LEADS TO
FURTHER COUGHING.
Ign. *428*.

< ON WAKING.
Lach. *497*, Kali bich. *458*.
Nux. v. *604*.

< EVERY MORNING.
Alum. *36*. Agar. *21*.

< DAILY AT 3 A.M.
Ammon. carb. *43*, Kali carb.
473.

< FIRST TAKING A BREATH.
Con. *323*.

< 11–12 P.M.
Hepar *406*.

< 2–5 A.M.
Kali carb. *471*.

< AT NIGHT.
Ammon. carb. *43*, Caps. *203*,
Hepar *406*. Hyos. *414*. Con.
327. Colch. *309*, Lyc. *581*, Pet.
631. Hyos. *411*.

< INHALING COLD AIR.
Rumex. Phos. *643*, Allium *32*.

< DRY COLD WEATHER.
  Caps. *203*, Hepar *403*.

< COLD DAMP.
  Phyt. *651*.

< CHANGE FROM WARM TO
  COLD.
  Phos. *643*.

< WARM OR COLD.
  Caps. *203*.

< DRAUGHTS.
  Caps. *203*, Hepar *403*.

< ENTERING WARM ROOM.
  Bry. *149*.

< LYING DOWN.
  Hyos. Puls *685*, Con. *327*.
  Hyos. *411. 414*.

> SITTING UP IN BED.
  Puls. *685*.

< LYING ON LEFT SIDE.
  Phos *643*.

< LYING ON RIGHT SIDE.
  Kali carb. *473*.

<LYING ON BACK.
  Agar. *21*.

< SITTING.
  Caps. *203*.

> SITTING UP.
  Hyos. *411. 414*.

> SITTING UP TO COUGH.
  Con. *323, 327*.

< SPEAKING.
  Bry. *149*.

< ON GETTING ANGRY.
  Ant. tart. *61*, Caps. *203*.

< FROM MENTAL EXCITEMENT.
  Cistus *287*.

< WARM DRINKS.
  Caps. *203*.

> DRINKING COLD WATER.
  Coccus. Cup. *345*.

< EATING OR DRINKING
  ANYTHING HOT.
  Mez. *554*.

< ON EATING.
  Ant. tart. *6*.

< ONIONS.
  Allium. *32*.

< EXHALING.
  Kreos. *480*.

> PRESSURE.
  Kreos *480*.

< SMOKING TOBACCO.
  Bry. *149*.

< BENDING FORWARD.
  Caust. *224, 228*.

WITH:
  stitches in sternum. Bry. *149*.
  internal heat. Bry. *149*.
  sensation of tightness or
  tension. Apis. *75*.

AFRAID TO COUGH BECAUSE
SOMETHING WILL BURST.
  Apis. *75*.

AFRAID TO COUGH FOR FEAR OF
A PAROXYSM.
  Cina *281*.

NO CHOKING WITH COUGH.
  Hepar. Brom. *139. 141*.

CRAMPS
  Abrot. *1, 2*, Cup. (Calc. *155*).

IN CALVES.
Camphor xv Anac. *48*, Cann. *189*. Calc. Cup. *345*.

IN CALVES FROM FEAR.
Lach. *499*.

IN ABDOMEN.
Canth. *198*.

IN MUSCLES.
Canth. *198*.

IN LEGS.
Canth. *198*, Cham. *241*.

IN FEET.
Caust. *229*. Cham. *241*.

IN NECK.
Cicuta *263*.

ON GETTING INTO COLD BED.
Calc. *155*.

ON STRETCHING LEGS IN BED.
Calc. Cup. *345*.

VIOLENT CRAMPS.
Cup. *345*.

OF WRITERS.
Mag. phos *526*.

OF PIANO AND VIOLIN PLAYERS.
Mag. phos. *526*.

FROM PROLONGED EXERTION.
Mag. phos *527*.

CRANIO-SPINAL AXIS
Cocc. *291*.

CRAVINGS
ACIDS.
Ant. tart. *66*, Cistus *287*, Carbo v. *209*, Kali bich. *459*.

Psor. *677*, Stram. *777*, Theridion. *816*

ALCOHOL.
Sul. *788*, Nux. v. *609*.

APPLES.
Ant. tart. *66. 69*.

BACON.
Calc. p. *166*, Mez. *546*, San. *733*.

BANANAS.
Theridion *816*.

BEER.
Kali bich. *459*, Nux. v. *609*.

BRANDY.
Theridion *816*.

BREAD.
Ferr. *372*.

BREAD IN MILK.
Abrot *1*.

CHALK.
Nitric ac. *591*.

CHEESE.
Arg. nit. Ast. r. Ign. Mosch. Puls. *Cistus 285*.

COFFEE.
Bry. *149*, Carbo v. *209*. Lach. *499*, Mez. *553*.

COFFEE AND TEA GROUNDS.
Alum. *35*, Con. *328*.

COLD WATER.
Tub. *837*. Ver. alb. *854*, Tarent. *800*.

EGGS
Calc. *154, 157. 161*. (Calc. p. *170*).

>EATING EGGS.
Calc. *157*.

FATS.
Ars. Hepar. Nux v. Sul. Nitric
ac. *586. 591*. Nux. v. *609*. San.
733. Sul. *786*.

FISH.
Nat. mur. *572*.

FRUITS.
Ant. tart. *66*, Cistus *287*, Ver.
alb. *854*.

FRUITS (GREEN).
Med. *531*.

FRUIT AND VEG. (EXCEPT
POTATOES).
Alum. *35*.

HAM.
Calc. p. *166. 170*. Mez. *546.
553*.

HERRINGS.
Nitric ac. *591*.

HOT DRINK.
Lyc. *515*.

ICES OR ICY DRINKS.
Med. *531*. Phos. *643*. Puls. *686*.
Ruta. *720* Ver. alb. *854*.

LIME.
Nitric ac. *591*.

LIQUORS.
Iod. *434*. Kreos. *480* Lach *499*.
San. *733*.

LIQUOR, ALTHOUGH
PREVIOUSLY DISLIKED.
Mez. *531*.

MEAT.
Iod *434*, Kreos. *480*. Lil. tig.
509.

MEAT, SALTED.
Calc. p. *166*, Mag. carb.
(Calc. p. *170*) San. *733*.

MILK.
Abrot. *1*. Mez. *546*, Nat. mur.
572. *Tub*. 837.

ONIONS.
Allium. *32*.

OYSTERS.
Lach. *499*. Nat. mur. *572*.

OYSTERS, BUT IS MADE ILL BY
THEM.
Lyc. *515*.

ORANGES.
Med. *531*. Theridion. *816*.

PASTRIES.
Puls. *686*.

PICKLES.
Hepar. *404*.

SALT.
Nat. mur. Phos. *641*. San. *733*.
Arg. nit. *82*. Carbo v. *209*.
Con. *328*. Med. *530*. Nat. mur.
570. 572. Sul. Nitric ac. *586*.

SUGAR.
Ammon carb. *42. Arg. nit. 79,
80*.

SUGAR, BUT CANNOT DIGEST IT.
Arg. nit. *79*.

SOUR THINGS.
Con. *328* Med. *531*. Nat. mur.
572.

SWEETS.
Arg. nit. Aeth. *17*. (Phos *643*)
Med. *531*, Carbo. v. *209*. Cina
281, Lyc. *515*, Sepia. *741*. Sul.
788.

TOBACCO.
Staph. *767*. Theridion. *816*.

VINEGAR.
Sepia *741*. Hepar *404/5*. Stram.
777.

WINE.
  Sepia *741*, Theridion. *816.*
  Aeth. *17*. Mez. *553.*

WHISKY.
  antidoted by Ledum. *504.*

INDIGESTIBLE THINGS.
  Alum. *35.*

STIMULANTS.
  Crot. *336, 339.*

SNOW.
  Crot casc. (Crot. *339*).

INCREDIBLE THINGS.
  Cycl. *351.*

SMOKING.
  antidoted by Caladium.
  (Ledum *504*).

LIGHT.
  Stram. *778.*

CROUP

**WITH NECK STRETCHED OUT,
HEAD BENT BACK.**
  Ant. tart. *66.*

CROUPY COUGH.
  Allium *31*, Iod. *434.*

GASPING AND CHOKING.
  Brom. *140. 141.*

INFLAMMATION OF WINDPIPE.
  Acon. *7.*

SUDDEN ATTACKS WITH:
  sudden difficulty in breathing.
  Acon. (Hepar *403*).
  hoarseness. Spongia. (Hepar *403*).
  suffocative cough. Hepar *403.*
  dry deep cough from difficulty in breathing. *Hepar 403.*
  rattling in chest. Hepar *407.*

MEMBRANOUS.
  Kali bich. *458*. Spongia (Hepar *403*).
  first inflammation. Acon. (Hepar *403*).
  followed by Spongia. (Hepar *403*).

AFTER EXPOSURE TO DRY COLD WINDS.
  Hepar *407.*

IN LIGHT HAIRED FAIR CHILDREN.
  Kali bich. *456.*

WAKES FROM SLEEP.
  Kali bich. *456.*

LARYNGISMUS STRIDULUS.
  Mag. phos. *525.*

CRURA CEREBRI
  Cocc. *291.*

CRUSTA LACTEA
  See SKIN.

CRUSTA SERPIGINOSA
  Calc. *160.*

CURE
DEFINITION OF . . .
  China *254.*

CYANOSIS
IN CHILDREN.
  Ant. tart. *61/2.*

AFTER LENGTHY DYSPNOEIA.
  Brom. *140.*

CYSTITIS

INFLMMATION OF MUCOUS MEMBRANES.
Ant. tart. *68.*

CYSTIC SWELLINGS.
Calc. *164.*

WITH SCALDING URINE.
Canth. 196.

D

DEBILITY

FEELS NOT AT ALL WELL, WITHOUT KNOWING WHAT IS THE MATTER.
Chel. *249.*

WEAKNESS IS THE MAIN SYMPTOM.
China *255/6*, Sil. *755.* Mur. ac. *564.*

WEAKNESS FROM:
loss of 'humours' China *255, 260.*
loss of blood. China *255, 259.*
loss of milk. China *255, 259.*
profuse sweats. China *255, 260.*
purgatives, diarrhoea. China *256. 259.*

AFTER:
flu. Chilly & weak. China *256.*
nerves or mental worries. Scut. (China *257*).
heaviness and shakiness. Gels. (China *257*).
unbearable tempers.

Influenzinum *200* C (China *257*).

loss of sleep. Cocc. *292*, Colch. *304.*

acute ailments. Psor. *673.*

FROM:
vomiting. Kali bich. *454.*
indigestion as result of loss of sleep. Colch. *304.*

OF SPINAL ORIGIN.
Cocc. *292.*

MUSCULAR.
Picric ac. *656.*

WITH FREQUENT DESIRE TO LIE DOWN.
Kali carb. *474.*

WITH HAEMORRHAGIC TENDENCY.
Kreos. *483.*

SO WEAK, SLIDES DOWN BED.
Mur. ac. *564.*

WITH WEAKNESS.
Phos. ac. (Picric ac. *655*)
Picric ac. *656.*

LETHARGY.
Chel. *249.*

ANAEMIC.
Ferr. phos. (China *256*).

NERVOUS.
Phos. ac. *639 (China 256)* Lyc. *519.*

< IN OPEN AIR.
Psor *673.*

INCREASING WITH ABDOMINAL AFFLICTIONS.
Psor. *677.*

DECUBITUS

PECULIAR POSITIONS TAKEN UP
IN BED.
Pet. *629*. Pyrogen. *695*.

DEGLUTITION

ACT OF SWALLOWING.
Bapt. *115*. Bell. *122*.

DELIRIUM

WILD MANIACAL.
Cup. *345*. Stram *772/3* Ver.
alb. *855*.

with considerable fever.
Stram. *772*.

with very little fever. Hyos.
(Stram. *772*).

with periodic fever. Bell.
(Stram. *772*).

VIOLENT.
1) Bell. *2*) Stram. *3*) Hyos.
Bell. *120, 116. 119*. Canth. *196*.

< at night. Ars. *98*.

DELIRIUM TREMENS (MANIA A
POTU).
Stram. *769, 774*. Agar. *24*. Arn.
88. Crot. *339*. Hyos. *409*. Kali
br. *467*, Opium. 614, Ran. b.
700.

IRRATIONAL.
Stram. *773*.

CONSTANT RAVING.
Ver. alb. *853*, Agar. *24*.

DELIRIOUS AT NIGHT.
Bapt. *114*.

LOQUACIOUS.
Crot. *336*, Lach. *499*.

WITH:
anxiety about the future. Bry.
147. Ver. alb. *853*.

anxiety about business. Bry.
147.

loss of decency. Hyos. Bell.
120.

pain. Ver. alb. *853*.

angular jerkings in . . . Hyos
(Stram *778*).

graceful rhythmical
movements in . . . Stram. *778*.

hallucinations. Stram. *773/4*.
Cann. *179*. Stram. *769*. Hyos
412. (cf. Agaricus, Bell.
Camph. Crocus).

hallucinations in the dark.
Stram. *774*.

with delusions. Hyos. Opium.
Stram. Pet. *629*.

delusions of elephants,
rhinoceri. Cann. *182*.

< WATER.
Stram. *773*.

HYDROPHOBIA.
Stram. *773*.

MUTTERING.
Ail. *26/7 29*. Bapt. *114*. Mur.
ac. *564*.

'BUSY' DELIRIUM OF EVERY
DAY BUSINESS.
Bry. Bell. *119*.

INCLINATION TO BITE THOSE
AROUND.
Bell. *120/1*.

MAY BE DELIRIOUS.
Ammon carb. *44*. Bapt. *112*.

KNOWS NOBODY.
Agar. *24*. Ail. *26*.

SINGS AND TALKS BUT WON'T
ANSWER.
Agar. *24*.

SEES ROLLING LIVE THINGS.
Cocc. *291*.

AT ONSET OF MENSES.
Cocc. *291*.

ON CLOSING EYES.
Pyrogen *691*.

STUPID, LAUGHS INCESSANTLY.
SAL. AC. *724*.

DEPRESSION

WITH CONSTANT WEEPING.
Apis. *74*. Lil. tig. *508*.

fits of uncontrollable weeping.
Kali br. *466*.

constant talking. Cimic. *275*.

suicidal ideas. Aurum. (Phos.
ac. *634*).

desire for suicide.
Ornithogalum. (Graph. *398*).

PROFOUND.
Kali br. *467*, Ornithogalum.
617. 618 Ptelea *679*.

MELANCHOLIA.
Kali br. *467*.

WITH FEAR OF DISEASE.
Lil. tig. *508*.

DESPONDENT.
Mez. *551*.

IN EVENING.
Nitric ac. *589*.

EXTREME INDIFFERENCE.
Phos. ac. *634*.

DIABETES. Rhus.
aromatica (Rhus. *716*)

WITH LUNG COMPLICATIONS.
Calc. p. *168*.

constant urging of urine. Nat.
phos. *578*.

constant craving for raw
articles. Tarent. *801*.

INSIPIDUS.
Phos. ac. *639*.

TRUE GLYCOSURIA.
Phos. ac. *639*.

DIARRHOEIA

GREENISH.
Arg. nit. Aeth. *17*. Cham. *240*.
Merc. *543*. Nat. phos. *576/7*.

ALTERNATELY GREENISH OR
YELLOWISH.
Dulc. *364. 366*.

YELLOW.
China *260*. Phos. ac. *638*.

WHITE.
Med. *535*. Phos. ac. *638*.

BLOODY.
Colch. *302*.

WATERY.
Ant. crud. *53*. Cham. *240*.
China *259*, Mur. ac. *564*. Nat.
mur. *572*. Phos. ac. *635*.

with much flatulence. Arg.
nit. *80*. China. *260*. Ferr. *370*.

LIKE JELLY.
Colch. *306*.

PAINLESS.
China. *259. 260*. Psor. *677*.
Stram. *770*, Sul. *788*.

CHANGEABLE.
San. *732.*

PROFUSE.
Phos. *643.* Ver. alb. *854.*

SUDDEN.
Camph. *173.* Phos. *645.*

VERY DEBILITATING.
China. *259.*

GUSHING.
Pet. *629.*

VIOLENT.
Canth. *193.* China *258.* Merc. cor. Lil. tig. *510.*

like spinach flakes. Arg. nit. *80.*

with vomiting. Kreos. *480.* Bapt. *112.* Cup. *343.*

PUTRID.
Kreos. *482.*

FETID, EXHAUSTING.
Bapt. *115.* Carbo. v. *211.* Cham. *240.* Graph. *395.*

SOUR SMELLING.
Calc. *159.* Cham. *240.* China. *259.* Nat. phos. *576.*

ODOUR – CARRION LIKE.
Psor *678,* Ptelea. *679.*

very offensive. Pyrogen. *696.*

SLIMY, WITH BELLYACHE.
Cham. *240.*

INVOLUNTARY.
Stram. *770.*

with anus wide open. Phos. Apis *75.* China. *259.*

CHRONIC.
Sul. *782.* Phos. *642.* Nat. sul. *585.*

of children. Collin. *311.*

AFTER RISING, REGULARLY.
Nat. sul. *580. 585.* Sul. *788.*

HURRIES FROM BED.
Sul. (Nat. sul. *580*).

< IN THE MORNING.
Bry. Nat. sul. *583. 585.*

< ON MOVING.
Bry. Nat. sul. *583.*

CHRONIC WITH EXCESSIVE SWEAT.
Tub. *837.* Ver. alb. *854.*

ALWAYS IN DAYTIME.
Pet. *629. 630.*

< DURING DAY.
Pet. *631.*

AFTER MIDNIGHT.
Sul. *788.*

IN MORNING.
Aloe. Sul. Tub. *837.*

COLICKY.
Coloc. (Kali carb. *471*). Mag. phos. *524.*

recurring. Kali carb. *471.* Ver. alb. *854.*

ALTERNATING WITH RHEUMATISM. Abrot. *2.*

ALTERNATING WITH CONSTIPATION.
Ant. crud. 54. 56. Chel. *251.* Cimic. *273.* Ptelea. *679.* Sul. *791.*

AFTER SUDDEN ATTACK.
Abrot. *2.* Camph. *173.* Nat. sul. *585.*

IN ANTICIPATION (BEFORE
EXAMINATIONS ETC.).
Gels. Aeth. *17*. Arg. nit. Gels.
383.

FROM EXCITEMENT.
Arg. nit. Gels. Phos. ac.
Thuja. Sil. *759*. Gels. *384*.

WITH DRY MOUTH.
Sul. *782*.

AFTER VEXATION, WITH
HEADACHE.
Calc. p. *168*.

WHENEVER URINATING.
Alum. *36*.

FEELING OF . . .
Ail. *28*.

BURNING.
< heat. Ars. *97*.

WITH:
headache in schoolgirls. Calc.
p. *166*. *168*.
burning. Canth. *193*.
much flatulence. Aloe, Calc.
phos. Nat. sul. *583*.
prolapse of rectum. Mur. ac.
564.
tenesmus, preceded by
griping pains. Ptelea. *679*.
restlessness. Pyrogen. *696*.
extreme violence of
evacuation. Ver. alb. *857*.
constant hunger. Pet. *631*.

FROM PANCREATIC
AFFECTIONS.
Iod. *434*.

IN PEOPLE WITH T.B. FAMILY
HISTORY.
Dros. *360*.

FOLLOWED BY HAMMERING IN
ANUS.
Lach. *498*.

RELIEF FROM . . .
Cimic *277*, Phos. ac. *635*.

OF OLD PEOPLE.
Ant. crud. *54*.

MAY BE BROUGHT ON BY
SMOKING.
Borax. *133*.

PRECEDED BY CUTTING IN
ABDOMEN.
Bry. *149*.

FROM JUICY FRUIT OR CIDER.
Calc. p. *168*.

OF UNDIGESTED FAECES.
China *258*. *260*.

< COLD WET WEATHER.
Rhod. *705*. Dulc. *363/4*.

< BEFORE A THUNDERSTORM.
Rhod. *705*.

< FROM VINEGAR, ACIDS, SOUR
WINE.
Ant. crud. *53*.

< FROM OVERHEATING.
Ant. crud. *53*.

< AFTER COLD BATHING.
Ant. crud. *53*.

< AT NIGHT AND EARLY
MORNING.
Ant. crud. *53*.

< ACID FRUITS.
Cistus *287*.

< FRUITS.
Cistus *287*.

< COFFEE.
Cistus *287*.

< EXCESS OF ACID.
Nat. phos. *576*.

< CABBAGE.
Pet. *629*.

< BEER.
Kali bich. *455*.

< OF AUTUMN.
Kali bich. *455*.

DIPHTHERIA

Brom. *140, 142*. Phyt. *649*. Iod. *433*. Mur. ac. *565*.

prophylactic *Lac. can. 487*.

'specific' *Merc. cy.* (Merc. *545*).

DIFFICULT BREATHING.
Apis. *74*.

SWOLLEN THROAT.
Apis *74*.

BEGINS ON LEFT SIDE.
Lach. *493*.

BEGINS ON RIGHT SIDE.
Lyc. *515, 520*.

'NEVER WELL SINCE' . . .
Lac. can. *489*.

MALIGNANT.
Crot. *336*. Tarent. *806*.

EPISTAXIS OF . . .
Crot. *337*.

IN FIRST STAGES.
Ferr. phos. *380*.

DARK OFFENSIVE BLOOD IN MENSTRUATION DURING . . .
Crot. *338*.

POST-DIPHTHERITIC PARALYSIS.
Gels. 382. Lac. can. *491*. Cocc. *294*. Plumbum *663*. Lyc. *515*.

< IN CHILDREN WITH FAIR SKINS.
Brom. *139*.

< AFTER SLEEP.
Lach. Ammon. carb. *46*.

WITH:
thick yellow membrane. Kali bich. *456. 458*.

stringy discharges. Kali bich. *456*.

fetor. Kreos. *478*. Merc. cor. (Lyc. *520*).

blue, dry, painful throat. Phyt. *652*.

tonsils swollen, covered with membrane, with white or yellow spots etc. Phyt. *652*.

restlessness. Rhus. *708*.

DISEASES

TWO SIMILAR DISEASES CANNOT:
suspend on another.

repel one another.

exist together to form a double complex disease. Thuja *823*.

INDEFINITE CHRONIC ILL-HEALTH.
Thuja *824*.

CHRONIC PARASITIC . . .
Thuja *825*.

'Thuja disease' Thuja *828*.

DISEASE AND DRUG SYMPTOMS.
China. *253*.

DIZZINESS
Ail *26*.

MUST SIT DOWN.
Alum. *36*.

CEREBRAL STATES — GIDDINESS OF ELDERLY PEOPLE.
Bellis *130*.

DOCTRINE OF SIGNATURES
Chel. *244. 246*. Hyp. *416*.

DREAMS
VIVID, OF DAY'S EVENTS.
Cicuta *263*.

VIVID, BUT UNREMEMBERED.
Cicuta *263*.

VIVID, CONFUSED.
Ruta. *722*, Sul. *791*.

HORRIBLE DREAMS OF CHILDREN.
Kali br. *467*, Sil. *751, 755*.

CHILD STARTS OUT OF SLEEP SCREAMING.
Calc. *154*.

AMOROUS, WITH SEMINAL EMISSIONS.
Staph. *764*.

OF:
climbing. Brom. *139*.
journeying. Brom. *139*.
quarrels. Brom. *139*, Bry. *147*, Nux. v. *609*.
fighting. Brom. *139*, Nux. v. *609*.
business. Bry. *148*.
robbers. Nat. mur. *572*.
snakes. Hyos. Lac. can. (Cann. *182*) Bell. Lac. can. *491*.
fire. Hepar. *406*.
urinating. Kreos. *480*, Sep. Lac. can. *491*.
lice. Nux. v. *609*.
being pursued, bitten by animals. Sul. *791*.
misfortune. Nux. v. *609*.
falling from height. Thuja *820*.
dead people. Thuja *820*.
water. Ver. vir. *862*.

DROPSY
Apis. 71. 73.

GENERAL ANASARCA.
Ars. *97*.

ASCITES.
Colch. *309*, Apis 71. Tereb. *812*.

AFTER HAEMORRHAGES OR EXCESSIVE LOSS OF FLUIDS.
China. *260*.

AFTER SCARLET FEVER.
Colch. *305*.

FROM CARDIAC DISEASE.
Collin. *311*.

OF ABDOMINAL CAVITY, PLEURAE, PERICARDIUM, SEROUS SACS.
Colch. *305. 309*.

ALWAYS WITH PALE URINE.
Colch. *305*.

ACUTE.
Colch. *308*.

WITH RENAL AFFECTIONS.
Colch. *308*.

HYDROTHORAX.
Colch. *309*.

WITH RED SAND IN URINE.
Lyc. *515*.

DROPSICAL LIMBS BECOME
FETID AND ULCEROUS.
Merc. *544*.

WITH THIRST.
Ars. *97*.

WITHOUT THIRST.
Apis, Ars. *97*.

DUVERNIS GLANDS
Borax. *136*.

DYNAMIZATION
Carbo v. *206*.

DYSENTERY
IN EARLY STAGES.
Ferr. phos. *379*.

CHRONIC.
Cistus *285*.

HAEMORRHOIDAL.
Collin. *311*.

AUTUMNAL.
Colch. *307*.

TYMPANIC.
Canth. Merc. Colch. *304*.

DIARRHOEIA OF . . .
Colch. *302*.

COLD AFTER EVERY DRINK.
Caps. *203, 205*.

OF SEPTIC ORIGIN.
Crot. *337*.

WITH:

ischura. Arnica *89*.

great tenesmus. Mer. cor
(Merc. *538*).

colic and fainting. Merc. *538*.

pain after stool. Nitric ac. *588*.

tenesmus all the time. Merc.
(Nitric ac. *588*).

violent cramps. Mag. phos.
527.

tearing pains down thigh
during stool. Rhus *708*.

dark stools. Rhus *708*.

no desire for stool. Nux. v.
606.

small and unsatisfactory
stools. Nux. v. *606*.

pain and strain continuing
after stool. Mer. cor. (Nux. v.
606). i.e. 'never-get-done'
sensation.

< COLD DAMP WEATHER.
Dulc. *365*.

> AFTER STOOL.
Nux. v. (Nitric ac. *588*) Nux v.
606.

< BY DAY.
Pet. *630*.

< COLD WET WEATHER.
Rhod. *705*.

< THUNDERSTORMS.
Rhod. *705*.

< EARLY MORNING.
Sul. *789*.

DYSMENORRHEA

PAINFUL MENSTRUATION. See
  FEMALE SEX.

DYSPEPSIA.
Nux. v. Anac. *50* (*200*th. per
Nash) Colch. *302*.

CHRONIC.
  Ptelea. *679*.

PAIN ONLY WHEN STOMACH IS
  EMPTY.
  Anac. 50.

PAIN RELIEVED BY EATING.
  Anac. *50*.

PAIN RELIEVED AFTER PROCESS
  OF DIGESTION IS OVER.
  Nux. v. Anac. *50*.

< 2–3 HOURS AFTER EATING.
  Anac. *50*.

> 2–3 HOURS AFTER EATING.
  Nux v. Anac. *50*.

DAILY SEVERE FLATULENCE.
  Puls. Carbo v. Arg. nit. *82*.

WITH PROLAPSUS ANI.
  Arn. *89*.

FROM TORPIDITY, ESPECIALLY
  IN OLD PEOPLE.
  Caps *201*.

WITH WATERBRASH AND
  HAEMORRHOIDS.
  Collin. *311*.

WITH BLOATING AFTER
  EATING.
  Kali carb. *471*.

OF AGED PERSONS INCLINED TO
  OBESITY.
  Kali carb. *472*.

DYSPNOEA

DIFFICULTY IN BREATHING.
  Verat. Ammon. carb. *46,*
  Hepar. *405*.

GREAT DYSPNOEA.
  Brom. *138,* Collin. *312*.

PAROXYSMAL.
  Ipec. *440*.

VIOLENT.
  Ipec. *445*.

SUFFOCATIVE.
  Camph. *174*. Ipec. *440*.

SPASMODIC.
  Asaf. *102*. Ipec. *440*. Cup. *343*.

HAS TO BE SUPPORTED TO SIT
  UP IN BED.
  Ant. tart. *69*.

DURING SLEEP.
  Lyc. *519*.

AS FROM CONTRACTION OF
  LUNGS.
  Mez. *553*.

AS IF CHEST MUSCLES FAIL TO
  ACT.
  Vib. *865*.

DURING DAMP, CLOUDY
  WEATHER.
  Nat. sul. *581/2 585*.

WITH:
  great sweating. Brom. *140*.

  continued yawning. Brom.
  139.

  cerebral congestion. Cimic.
  273.

  exhausting from exertion.
  Calc. Cistus *287*. Lyc. *519*.

  palpitations. Ferr. *372*. Psor.
  677.

feeling of weight on chest.
Nux. mosch. *597*.

< ON MOTION, ESPECIALLY
ASCENDING.
Ars. *96*.

E

EARS
Caust. *226*, Puls. Kali sul. *476*,
Med. *530*, Mur. ac. *563*.

DEAFNESS:
preceded by
oversensitiveness. Sul. *787*.
for human voice. Sul. *787*.
< after eating. Sul. *787*.
< blowing nose. Sul. *787*.
with noises near. Sal. ac. *724*.
from paralysis of auditory
nerve. Caust. *224*. Hyos. *413*.
in right ear. Ant. crud. *55*.
dating back to past Kerion
(suppurating form of
ringworm) Mez. *553*.
< riding in carriage. Graph.
Nitric ac. *590*.
with induration of tonsils.
Nitric ac. *590*.
after abuse of mercury. Nitric
ac. *590*.
syphilitic. Nitric ac. *590*.

OTITIS – INFLAMMATION.
Caps. *199*, Ferr. phos. *380*,
Mur. ac. *563*. Picric. ac. *656*.
lancinating, stinging pain.
Sul. *787*.

< by all noises. Sul. *787*.
chronic. Sul. *787*.

OTALGIA. – EARACHE.
Cham. *219*, Ferr. phos. *379*.
Mag. phos. *524*. Puls. Cham.
Allium *31*. Borax. *133*.
< at night. Dulc. *366*.

OTORRHEA – DISCHARGE FROM
EAR.
Calc. *160*. Elaps (Crot *357*)
Graph *395*. Cistus *287*, Calc.
160. Hepar *404*.
stinging, purulent discharge.
Kali bich. *456*.
with loss of hearing. Lyc. *517*.
offensive. Merc. *539*. Hepar.
404.

DISCHARGE OF STICKY
SUBSTANCE.
Graph. San. *733*.

YELLOW DISCHARGES.
Kali bich. *453*. *457*.

BLOODY DISCHARGES.
Asaf. *105*. Crot. *335*.

FETID OR PURULENT
DISCHARGES.
Asaf. *103*, Psor. *677*.

CHRONIC SUPPURATION.
Kali bich. *457*.

MENIERE'S DISEASE.
Sal. ac. *724*. (Sepia *746*).
Theridion *818*. Sal. ac. Rhod.
705.

TINNITUS.
Rhod. *705*.
roaring. Merc. *541*. Nitric ac.
590. Pet. *633*. Theridion *816*.

Cycl. *351*. Ant. crud. *55*.
Cham. *239*. Chel. *250*. Lyc.
517. Ledum *505*. Cycl. *351*.
ringing. Cann. *182*. China *260*.
Cycl. *351*.
buzzing. Cann. *182*.

BURNING, ITCHING, REDNESS.
Agar. *24*.

REDNESS WITH SORENESS
BEHIND.
Pet. *633*.

HOT AND RED.
Alum. *37*, Pyrogen *691*.

ITCHING.
Ammon carb. *42*. Caps. *200*.
Ign. *430*. Pet. *631*.

TEARING, ZYGOMA INTO EAR.
Lach. *497*.

DULLNESS AS FROM COTTON
WOOL IN EARS.
Cycl. *351*.

SENSATION OF WIND IN . . .
Mez. *551*.

NAUSEA FELT IN . . .
Dioscor. (Cocc. 298) Dulc.
361.

SCRATCHING PRESSURE IN . . .
Ruta *720*.

AUDITORY NERVE VERTIGO.
Sal. ac. *726*.

SORENESS BEHIND EARS.
San. *733*.

ITCHING BEHIND EARS.
Theridion. *816*.

SCURF ON OR BEHIND EARS.
Psor. *676*.

MOIST AND SORE PLACES
BEHIND EARS.
Graph. *399*. *400*.

OOZING ERUPTIONS BEHIND
EARS.
Mez. *556*.

PAIN AS FROM A BLOW.
Ruta. *720*.

STITCHING PAIN.
movement. Bry *144*. Chel. *250*.

PAIN DEEP IN EAR.
Caps. *200*. Cycl. *350*.

PAIN WITH EVERY COUGH.
Caps. *202*.

CRAMP-LIKE TWITCHING IN
EXTERNAL EAR.
Cina. *282*.

MEMBRANE TYMPANI
PERFORATED.
Kali bich. *457*.

POLYPS OF MEATUS.
Kali sul. *476*.

ACCUMULATION OF EAR WAX.
Con. *327*.

RESULT OF SUPPRESSED
ERUPTIONS.
Mez. *556*.

HEARS BETTER IN A NOISE.
Graph. *399*.

SENSATION OF A PLUG IN EAR.
Anac. *49*.

HARD OF HEARING FROM
CONCUSSION.
Arn. *88*.

BOILS IN EXTERNAL EAR.
Picric ac. *656*.

ONIONS IN EARS FOR EARACHE.
Puls. Allium *30, 32*.

COLD.
Carbo v. *207*.

ACUTE MIDDLE EAR DISEASE.
Bell. *117*.

INFLAMMATION OF OUTER EAR.
Calc. *160*. Merc. *541*.

INFLAMMATION OF INNER EAR.
Calc. *160*.

ULCERATION.
Calc. *160*.

MASTOIDS:
threatened. Hepar *404* (use CM).

swelling, periostitis, caries. *Caps. 199, 200, 202, 205*.

pressure under . . . Cina *282*.

fever after mastoid operation. Caps. *205*.

ECCHYMOSES
COLLECTION BENEATH SKIN OF BLOOD AS RESULT OF A BRUISE. See SKIN and STOMACH.

ECLAMPSIA
CONVULSIONS IN PREGNANCY — See CONVULSIONS.

ECPTYSIS
Merc. *542*.

ECZEMA
Colch. *302*. Ran. b. *700*. Rhus div. (Rhus *716*).

RAW, EXCORIATED.
Rhus. *715*.

BURNING.
Rhus. *715*.

INCESSANT ITCHING.
Rhus. *715*.

INTOLERABLE ITCHING.
Mez. *552*. Rhus. *715*.

DRY, OF CHILDREN.
Calc. s. *172*.

COPIOUS EXUDATION.
Mez. *552*.

IMPETIGINOUS (CRUSTA LACTEA).
Calc. s. *172*.

OF:
legs. Graph. *395*. Pet. *629*.

head (Excema capitis) Cicuta *261*, Graph. *396. 398*. Pet. *629*. Mez. *553*. Psor. *676*. < winter. Pet. *629*.

lids. eruptions moist. Graph. *396*. covered with crusts. Graph. *396*. very red. Sul. (Graph *396*).

ears. Lyc. *517*, Pet. *629*. Psor. *676*.

arms. Pet. *629*, Psor. *676*.

WITH:
hard horny scales. Ant. crud. Ran. b. *702*.

yellow moisture under crusts. Staph. *761*.

acid symptoms. Nat. phos. *576*.

AS RESULT OF SUPPRESSION.
Mez. *556*.

LUNG TROUBLES FROM ˙
SUPPRESSED ECZEMA.
Ars. *97.*

DURING WINTER, GETTING
BETTER IN SUMMER.
Pet. 630.

AS RESULT OF VACCINATION.
Thuja 822.

< FROM WARM APPLICATIONS.
Psor. *673.*

< AT NIGHT.
Psor *673.*

> FROM AIR.
Psor *673.*

(N.B. NORMAL PSOR.
reaction is < from open air).

EMACIATION

RAPID.
Ars. *97*, Ferr. *373*, Kreos. *478.*
482. Iod. Kreos. *483.*
with ravenous appetite. Iod.
Brom. *138.* Sil. *756.* Tub. *835.*

GREAT EMACIATION.
Nat. mur. *573.* Pet. *631.* Phos.
ac. *635.* Phos. *646.*

PROGRESSIVE.
San. *736.* Sil. *755.*

EVERYWHERE, EXCEPT
ABDOMEN.
Calc. *161.*

OF BODY, WITH ENLARGED
ABDOMEN.
Abrot. Nat. mur. Sul. Calc.
Iod. Sil. *756.* Sul. *788.*

WITH PROFOUND DEBILITY.
Iod. *433.*

Kreos. *480.* Tub. *837.*

EMACIATED CHILDREN.
Calc. p. *165.* Caust. *222.* San.
733. Calc. p. (Ferr. phos. *375*).

FROM ANAEMIA.
Plumbum. *669.*

WITH FALSE PLETHORA.
Ferr. *373.*

WITH GLANDULAR
ENLARGEMENT.
Iod. *432.*

EMACIATES ABOVE, WITH
EXTREMITIES WELL
NOURISHED.
Lyc. *521.* Nat. mur. *569.*

OF SUFFERING PARTS.
Ledum. *507. Plumbum. 663.*
669. Graph. *400.*

FROM CONTINUED VOMITING.
Kali bich. *454.*

IF > AT THE SEASIDE.
Med. *530.*

EMPHYSEMA
Ammon carb. *43*, Ant. tart. *66,*
68.

WITH BRONCHITIS.
Ledum. *502.*

ENCEPHALITIS
INFLAMMATION OF THE BRAIN.
See BRAIN.

ENTERALGIA
COLIC. See COLIC.

ENTERIC FEVER
Morb. *559.*

ENTROPION
LASHES TURNED IN. See EYES.

ENURESIS
San. *737*, San. (Cina *284*).

WITH GENERAL DEBILITY.
Calc. p. *168*.

DURING FIRST SLEEP.
Caust. *230*, Kreos. *480. 482. 484*.

NOCTURNAL, FROM NERVOUS IRRITATION.
Mag. phos. *525*.

WITH STRONG SMELLING URINE.
Med. *531*.

AS RESULT OF DRINKING TURPENTINE.
Tereb. *811*.

NIGHT OR DAY.
Tereb. *811*.

NOCTURNAL, NOT NECESSARILY CONNECTED WITH WORMS.
Cina *284*.

EPIGLOTTIS
Bell *122*.

EPILEPSY
Aeth. *18*. Anac. *50*. Mag. phos. *525*. Thuja *825*.

PETIT MAL.
Caust. *223*. Cicuta. *265. 269*. Viscum. *867* Nux. mosch *600*. Sil. *757*.

WITH:
convulsions. *Plumbum. 667*. Bell. *123*. Cicuta *263*.

stiffness of whole body. Aeth. *20*.

violent spasms. Aeth. *20*, Hyos. *414*.

vertigo. Calc. *159. 162*.

loss of consciousness. Calc. *162*.

pharyngeal spasms. Calc. *162*.

spasms starting in fingers and toes. Cup. *342*.

spasms of larynx. Bell. (Hyos *409*).

exaltation of all powers of body and mind. Cann. *180*.

swelling of stomach. Cicuta *264*.

thumbs turned inward. Cicuta. *264*.

purple face. Hyos. *409, 414*.

projecting eyes. Hyos. *409. 414*.

enuresis. Hyos. *409, 414*.

clutching of throat. Bell. (Hyos. *409*).

sardonic laughter. Stram. (Hyos. *409*).

stupid friendly look. Stram. (Hyos. *409*).

quick thrusting of head to right. Stram. (Hyos. *409*).

BEGINNING IN LOWER PART OF CHEST. *Cup. 344*.

FROM FRIGHT.
Caust. *223*.

FROM BEING CHILLED.
Caust. *223*.

WITH SENSATION OF MOUSE
RUNNING UP LEG.
Bell. Sil. Calc. *155*.

RESULT OF SOME VEXATION.
Ign. *425*.

RESULT OF SOME GREAT
FRIGHT.
Ign. *425*. Stram. *769*.

RESULT OF QUININE POISONING.
Nat. mur. *571*.

IN A 'SULPHUR' PATIENT.
Sul. *785*.

< DURING NIGHT.
Calc. *163*.

< DURING SOLSTICE AND FULL
MOON.
Calc. *163*.

< SLIGHTEST TOUCH OR JAR.
Cicuta. *264:*

< MENSES.
Cimic. *276*.

EPISTAXIS
NOSEBLEED.
Caps. *200*, Vipera. Ferr. phos.
380. Acon. *9*. Ant. crud. *55*.
Arn. *87*. Hepar. *405*. Nitric ac.
593.

CHRONIC.
Vipera. Bry. *147*.

PROFUSE.
Crot. *335*.

THIN, UNCOAGULABLE.
dark. Crot. *336*.

CLEAR HOT BLOOD.
Dulc. *363*.

VICARIOUS MENSTRUATION.
Bry. *147*.

IN MORNING.
Bry. *148*.

FROM MECHANICAL CAUSES.
Arn. *87*.

WHEN WASHING FACE.
Ammon. carb. *43*.

< AFTER GETTING WET.
Dulc. *363*.

IN NERVOUS CHILDREN.
Ferr. *370*.

DURING SLEEP.
, Merc. *541*.

WITH:
bright red blood. Ipec. *444*.
imaginary smells. Puls. Kali
sul. *476*.
swollen, dry nose. Phos. *645*.
dark coagulated blood. Plat
660.
stuffed coryza. Puls. *684*.
dark clots. Tarent. *799*.

EPITHELIOMA
MALIGNANT TUMOUR IN THE
SKIN. See SKIN.

ERETHISM
EXCITEMENT OR STIMULATION
OF AN ORGAN, ABNORMAL
IRRITABILITY.
Ferr. *371*. Hyos. *409*.

ERUCTATIONS
BELCHING. See
FLATULENCE.

ERYSIPELAS

INFLAMMATION OF THE SKIN, WITH FEVER. See SKIN.

ESCHAROTIC

POWERFUL CAUSTIC.
Kali bich. *455.*

EXANTHEMA

ACUTE INFECTIOUS ERUPTIONS.
Ran. b. *700,* Pet. *629.*

EXOPHTHALMIA

PROTRUSION OF EYEBALLS. See EYES.

EYES

PUPILS:
dilated. Sul. (Calc. *160*). Con. *331.* Cycl. *350.* Hyos. *413.* Ipec. *444,* Ledum. *505.* Opium. *616,* Staph. *762,* Stram. *771, 774.* Ver. vir. *860.* Tarent *802.* Bell. *117. 121/2. 124.* Cicuta *262.* Cina *280.*
pain in . . . Cimic. *272. 275.*
hurt. Calc. p. *167/8.* Caps. *199.* Cimic. *271.*
contracted. Cicuta *262,* Opium. *616.*

EYEBALL:
pain in . . . Phos ac. *637,* Coloc. *318.*
bruised. Symphitum *200* C (Ledum *504*). Tub. *837.*
feel too large. Nat. mur. *574.*
'black eyes', blows on eyeballs. Symphitum *794.*

Ledum *504/5* (*200* C).

EYEBROWS — SPASMS IN.
Cina *282.*

SCLEROTICS, YELLOW.
Chel. Kali bich. *453,* Crot. *335.*

CORNEA:
pustules on. Calc. *160.*
abscesses of . . . Calc. sul. *172.*
dimness of . . . Calc. *160.*
opacity of . . . Arg. nit. *79,* Asaf. *102.*
ulcers on . . . Con. *327.* Kali bich. *459.*
keratitis — inflammation of . . . Sul. *787.*
ulceration of . . . in children. Tub. *834.*

DRY.
Alum. *36.* Bell. *122.* Mez. *551.* Nux. mosch. *596.*

RED HOT.
Glon. *389.* San. *733.*

BURNING.
Allium *31,* Alum. *36.* Ammon. carb. *42.* Con. *327.* Sul. *782.* Paeonia. *622.* Kreos *483.* Cycl. *349.* Puls. *683.* Sepia *743.* Caust *226.* Ars. *94. 98.* Caps. *199.* Bell. *122.* Ferr. phos. *380.*

BLEEDING.
Ail. *28.* Arn. *88.* Ledum. *504.*

INFLAMED.
Alum. *36/7.* Ant. crud. *52/3* Arn. *88.* Borax. *132.* Calc. *162.* Canth. *197.* Rhus. *712.* Arg. nit. Ruta. *718.* Carbo. v. *212.*

Caps. *199*. Ferr. phos. *380*.
Tub, Hepar *404*.

OEDAMATOUS.
Ars. *98*, Cham. *239*.

CONGESTED.
Ail. *28*.

PAIN IN . . . < MOTION.
Bry. *143*. *148*. Lyc. *516*. Ipec.
440.

STITCHING PAINS . . .
< MOVEMENT.
Bry. *144*.

ACHING PAIN IN . . .
Caps *200*.

PAIN OVER LEFT EYE.
Chel. *249*.

neuralgia in . . . Thuja. *823*,
Glon. *390*.

neuralgia in and over right
eye. Sang. *729*.

post orbital neuralgia, as
result of vaccinations. Thuja
822.

WATER PROFUSELY.
Allium. *30/2*. Med. *534*. Merc.
541.

CANNOT STAND LIGHT.
Allium. *30*.

PAROXYSMIC FLICKERING
BEFORE EYES.
Theridion. *816*.

SPOTS BEFORE . . . DARK.
Sul. *787*.

SICKLY ROUND . . .
Cina. *282*.

SPARKS BEFORE . . .
Ant. tart. *69*, Mag. phos. *524*.

BLUENESS ROUND . . .
Crot. *336*.

CLUSTERS OF RED VESSELS.
Arg. nit. *80*..

ROLLING OF EYES WITH EYES
CLOSED.
Cocc. *298*.

AGGLUTINATED.
Rhus. *712*.

< AT NIGHT.
Alumina. *35*. Lyc. *516*.

DIM AND FATIGUED FROM TOO
MUCH READING OR FINE
WORK.
Ruta *718*. *720*.

ITCHING.
Pet. *631*, Puls. *683*.

TWITCHING.
Cham. *241*, Cina *280*. Cup.
345.

AS IF PULLED OUTWARDS.
Con. *328*.

WEAKNESS IN . . .
Con. *327*.

STITCHES IN . . .
Lach. *499*. Nitric ac. *590*.

STYES IN . . .
Graph. *397*.

SMOKY APPEARANCE
BEFORE . . .
Gels. *385*.

CICATRICES ON EYE AFTER
OPERATION.
Graph. *397*.

FEEL TOO LARGE.
Plumbum. *670*.

LACHRYMATION.
Ruta. *720.*
with acrid excoriating tears.
Sul. *787.* Ars. *93. 98.* Nux. v.
604.
burning. Nat. sul. *584.*
by day. Alum. *36.* Bry. *148.*
Sepia *740.*

PAROXYSMS OF NYCTALOPIA.
Sul. *787.*

AS IF VEIL OR GAUZE BEFORE
EYES.
Sul. *787.*

PURULENT DISCHARGE FROM
EYES.
Arg. nit *79.* Hepar *404.* Merc.
541.

PURULENT OPHTHALMIA.
Arg. nit. *79.*

NUMBNESS ROUND EYE.
Asaf. *102.*

EXOPHTHALMOS.
Dros. *359.*

WATERY BLOODY FLUID.
Canth. *195.*

COLD FEELING BEHIND EYES.
Calc. p. *167.*

PRESSURE FROM WITHIN
OUTWARDS.
Aur. *110.* Cham. *239.* Cimic.
273. Ferr. *372.*

VERY ENLARGED BLOOD
VESSELS.
Aesc. *16.*

CONJUNCTIVITIS.
Ant. tart. *68.* Colch. *302.*
Hepar. *406.* Nat. sul. *584.* Pet.
633.

CONJUNCTIVA PUCKERED.
Arg. nit. *80.*

CHEMOSIS — SWELLING OF
CONJUNCTIVAL MEMBRANE.
Arg. nit. *79.*

WEAKNESS OF INTERNAL
RECTUS.
Alum. *39.*

LETTERS RUN TOGETHER.
Cann. *182.* Nat. mur. *572.*
Ruta. *720.*

DIPLOPIA — DOUBLE VISION.
Con, *322,* Gels. *383. 385.*
Graph. *397.* Aur. *110.* Nitric
ac. *590.*

CATARACT INCIPIENT.
Caust. *226,* Chel. *244.*
Ammon. carb. *42.*
CATARACT.
Sul. *787.*

AMBLYOPIA.
Cina *284.*

ATROPHY OF OPTIC DISC.
Cina *284.*

CHOROIDITIS.
Cina. *284.*

COLDNESS IN EYES.
Ammon. carb. *42.*

COLDNESS, CRAWLING IN EYES.
Plat. *662.*

CATARRHAL, ULCERATIVE.
Arg. nit. *79.* Asaf. *102.*

EYESTRAIN.
Nat. mur. Senega. Ruta *719*
Ruta. Symphitum. *794.*

GLAUCOMA.
Sul. *787.*

LOSS OF SIGHT FROM
HAEMORRHAGES.
China 260.

MACULAE.
Calc. 160.

OPACITY.
Calc. 160.

OPHTHALMIA.
Calc. 160. Apis. 75, Nat. mur.
572. Nitric ac. 590. Thuja 828.

PHOTOPHOBIA.
Calc. 160, Acon. 9.
Ail. 27. Caust. 226. Phos. 645.
Con. 324. Sepia 740. Nat. sul.
585. San. 737.

RETINITIS.
Cina. 282.

RETINAL ANAESTHESIA.
Cina 284.

STRABISMUS — SQUINTING.
Cicuta 262. Cycl. 350. Mag.
phos. 525, 527. Nat. phos. 576.

TRACHOMA.
Apis. 75.

SECRETION OF MEIBOMIAN
GLANDS.
Chel. 250.

YELLOW HALO ROUND LIGHT.
Alum. 36.

CHRONIC
BLEPHAROPHTHALMIA OF
CHILDREN.
Ant. crud. 53.

ASTHENOPIA.
Ruta. 720. Sepia. 740.

RECURRENT STYES.
Staph. 762.

SWELLING ON RIGHT
LACHRYMAL GLAND.
Sil. 753.

HALF SIGHT — UPPER OBJECTS
REMAIN INVISIBLE.
Aur. 110.

TENSION IN EYES INTERFERING
WITH VISION.
Aur. 110.

DAMAGE DUE TO INJURIES.
Arn. 88.

VISUAL DISTURBANCE WITH
HEADACHE.
Nat. phos. 578.

GONORRHEAL INFECTIONS OF
EYES.
Syph. Med. 530.

APOPLEXY OF RETINA.
Glon. 393.

COLOURS AND BRIGHT SPOTS
BEFORE EYES.
Kali bich. 472.

SQUINTING AFTER
CONVULSIONS.
Hyos. 413.

ABILITY TO SEE IN THE DARK.
Ferr. 372.

PUFFINESS BETWEEN
EYEBROWS AND LIDS.
Kali carb. 472.

FEEL AS IF EYES WERE FORCED
OUT WHEN THROAT WAS
PRESSED.
Lach. 497. 499.

MISTY EYES.
Merc. 541.

70

EYES DRAWN BACKWARD.
Mez. *554*.

ORBITAL CELLULITIS.
Rhus. 710.

< STOOPING.
Ferr. phos. *380*.

< VERY BRIGHT LIGHT.
Glon. *393*. Merc. *541*.

< HEAT.
Arg. nit. *79. 80*.

> HEAT.
Mag. phos. *527*.

< COLD.
Arg. nit. *79. 80*.

< LIGHT.
Calc. *160*. Con. *322. 327*.

< MORNING.
Calc. *160*.

< CHANGE OF WEATHER.
Calc. *160*.

YELLOW EYES.
Chel. *247, 250*.

EYELIDS:
blepharitis. Graph. *397*, Merc. *541*, Staph. *762*.

styes on . . Lyc. *516*.

open with difficulty. Con. *328*.

upper lids as if paralysed. Caust. Sep. Alum. *37*. Nitric ac. *590* Plumbum *670*, Sepia *743*.

fester and become cracked. Ammon. carb. *45*.

red, inflamed. Graph. Sul. *782*, Ant. crud. *52/3* Graph. *395. 399* Lyc. *516*. Kreos. *483*. Pet. *633*. Ruta *718*. Rhus. *712*.

Tub. *834*.

spasms of . . Ruta *720*. Calc. p. *168*.

ptosis - drooping of upper eyelids. Caust. Alum. *35*, Gels. Cocc. *294* Alum. *37*, Con. *322*. Mag. phos. *525*. Med. *530*. Ferr. *371* Con. *323, 327, 331*. Gels. *382. 385*. Nat. sul. 584.

from coughing. Nitric ac. *592*. Sepia *739/40*.

red. Sul. (Graph *397*) Lyc. *516*. Merc. *541*.

pale. Graph. *397*.

pain in . . Cimic. *271*, Ruta *718*.

paralysis of . . Caust. *226*. Con. *331*.

swelling of . . Cycl. *350*. Kreos. *478*. Rhus. *712*.

epithelioma of . . Con. *323*.

crack and bleed. Graph. *397*.

spasmodically close. Ars. (Graph. *397*) Nat. mur. *572*.

twitching. Mez. *546. 551*.

eczema of . . Mez. *553*.

pressure and smarting in . . Ran. b. *698*.

as if too heavy to open. Sepia *743*.

pressure on . . Staph. *762*.

CANTHI:
red. Arg. nit. *80*.

itching at inner canthus. Alum. *36/7*.

gum on outher canthi. Ipec.
444.

as if tightly compressed from
all sides. Cham. *239*. Lach.
497.

soreness of outer canthi. Ant.
crud. *53*.

pain in inner canthi. Staph.
762.

inflammation of external
canthi. Graph . . Graph. *399*.

EYELASHES
   entropion. Borax. *132. 136*,
   Graph. *397*.

WILD STARING LOOK.
   Stram. *774*.

STARING LOOK.
   Bell. *121*. Cann. *182/3* Cicuta
   264. Iod. *432*. Glon. *390* mag.
   phos. *525*. Mur. ac. *564*.
   Opium. *613*.

SUNKEN LOOK.
   Crot. *336*. Dros. *361*.

PROMINENT.
   Caps. *202*. Dros. *359*. Ferr.
   370. Glon. *393*. Iod. *433 436*
   Ver. alb. *856*.

FEELING EYES WILL BE
PRESSED OUT.
   Bell. *119*. Glon. *390*. Sang. *729*.

SMARTING.
   Sul. *787*. Alum. *36*. Kreos. *483*.
   Nitric ac. *590*.

VISION:
   dizzy, confusing. Theridion.
   816.
   dim. Cycl. *349*.

dazzling before eyes. Nat.
mur. *574*.

objects 'flicker'. Cycl. *349. 350*.

objects look red. Con. *322. 327*.
Bell. Hyos. *415*.

objects look striped. Con. *322.
327*.

objects look black. Stram.
(Hyos. *415*).

sees firey spots. Alum. *37*,
Psor. *676*. Sepia *740*.

sees firey zigzags. Nat. mur.
574. Sepia. *740*.

sees zigzag wreath of colours.
Nat. mur. Graph. Sepia *740*.

indistinct. Anac. *48*. Calc. p.
167. Cina *280*. Cocc. *296*. Gels.
385.

eyes close involuntarily.
Caust. *224*.

objects look very yellow. Kali
bich. *459*.

F

FACE
RED.
   Cicuta. *263*, Cina *281*. Camph.
   176. Acon. *11*. Ail. *26*. Bell.
   117, 122. Bry. *148. 150*. Cina
   282. Opium. *613*. Caps. *204*.
   Crot. *336*. Glon. *394*. Pyrogen.
   691.

RED, WITH LINEA NASALIS.
   Aeth. *18*.

DARK MAHOGANY.
   Ail. *27/9*. Carbo. v. *207*.

PURPLE.
Lach. *492*. Glon. *394*. Ail. *28*.
Ant. tart. *61*. Carbo. v. *207*.

BLUISH.
Ant. tart. *61,* Asaf. *104*.
Camph. *177*. Cimic. *276*. Cup.
345. Ver. alb. *856*.

VENOUS PURPLE.
Asaf. *104*.

DARK RED.
Bapt. *113, 115*. Cimic. *273*.

ROSY, BUT COLD.
Caps. *204*.

YELLOW.
Chel. *250*. Crot. *333*. Kreos.
483. Med. *534*. Ptelea *680*.
Sepia *740*.

YELLOW SADDLE ACROSS
BRIDGE OF NOSE.
Sepia. *740*.

FIERY RED WITH VERTIGO,
RINGING IN EARS,
PALPITATIONS, DYSPNOEA.
Ferr. *372*.

FLORID.
Ferr. phos. *380,* Opium *613,*
Tub. *837*.

FLUSHED, PLETHORIC.
Ferr. *373*. Sul. *791*.

FLUSHED FROM RUSH OF BLOOD
TO FACE.
Graph. *396*. Stram. *774*. Sul.
791.

RED, DURING CHILL.
Ign. *425*.

REDDISH BLOTCHES.
Kreos. *483*. Nat. phos. *576*.

FLUSHED HOT.
Glon. Bell. *117*. Cocc. *296. 298,*
Ferr. *373*. Sang. *729*. Glon.
394. Gels. *384/5*.

PALE AND SUNKEN.
Hyos. Bell. *120,* Cina. *281*.
Lyc. *520*.

PALE.
Borax. *133,* Calc. *159*. Calc. p.
168, China *260*. Cina *281/2*
Camph. *177*. Carbo v. *210*.

SALLOW.
Bapt. *115*. Calc. p. *168*. Lyc.
520. Plumbum. *668*.

PALE AND SICKLY, EYES
SUNKEN WITH DARK RINGS.
Ant. tart. *63, 66*.

SICKLY GREY ASH-COLOURED.
Brom. *140*.

DEATHLY.
Ars. *98*.

CADAVEROUS AND COLD.
Carbo v. *207, 210*.

CADAVERIC.
Colch. *304*.

LOOKS OLD.
Calc. *160*.

YELLOWISH-GREY.
Lyc. *517*.

GREASY.
Nat. mur. *569*.

PALE, EARTHY HUE.
Tarent. *799,* Ver. alb. *853*.

PALE, WITH PURPLE NECK.
Tarent *802*.

PALE, BUT EASILY FLUSHING.
Ferr. *370*.

CHANGES COLOUR VERY OFTEN
WHEN AT REST.
Ign. *425.*

WAXY LOOKING AS IF GREASED.
Thuja *820.*

ALTERNATE PALE AND RED
CHEEKS.
Sul. *791.*

HOT FLUSHES WITH FAINTNESS.
Sul. *791.*

GREASY.
Nat. mur. *569.*

ONE CHEEK HOT, ONE COLD.
Acon. *11.* Arn. *90. Cham 236/7
239, 242.*

BESOTTED.
Ail *28,* Asaf. *104.* Bapt. *113.
115.*

RATHER STUPID DULL FACE.
Sepia *747.*

ITCHY, PIMPLY.
Graph. *400.*

BARBER'S ITCH.
Cicuta. *265.*

PUSTULAR ERUPTIONS.
Cicuta. *263.*

WARTS ON . . .
Caust. *227.*

SKIN TENSE.
Alum. *37.*

WITH ERUPTIONS ON CHEEKS.
Ant. crud. *53,* Cicuta *263.*

HEAT OF FACE:
with cold hands. Dros. *361.*
with chills down back. Asaf.
26.

< EXPOSURE TO COLD.
Agar. *25.*

WITH COLD SWEAT.
Carbo v. *210.*

SWEATS AFTER EATING OR
DRINKING.
Cham. *239. 240.*

COLDNESS, CRAWLING AND
NUMBNESS IN R. SIDE OF . . .
Plat. *661.*

FOREHEAD, PRESSURE.
Phyt. *653*

NUMBNESS.
Glon. *388. 390.*

SAGGY LOWER JAW.
Gels. *385.*

BURNING:
dry heat in evening. Acon. *110*
cheeks and face. Ptelea *680.*

HEAT OVER WHOLE OF THE
FACE.
Cina *282.* Paeonia *622.* Sul.
782.

BURNING ON CHIN AND UPPER
LIP.
Ant. crud. *55.*

SWOLLEN.
Ail *28.* Ars. *98.* Bell. *122.* Kali
carb. *472.* Rhus. *712.* Crot.
336.

PUFFY.
Merc. *545.* Ver. alb. *856.* Bry.
148. Sepia *747.* Calc. *159. 160.*
Ferr. *373.* Ledum. *502.*

PAIN:
in jaws. Caust. *227,* Med. *534.*
arthritic in jaws. Caust. *227.*

in frontal sinuses. Sang. *730.*

at root of nose. Sang. *730.*

neuralgia of face. Ars. *95,*
Sang. *729.*

> pressing head firmly
against floor. Sang. *731.*

in skin above eyebrows. Coloc
318

distorted with pain. Coloc.
316.

JAWS:

caries of lower jaw. Cistus.
288.

trismus – lockjaw. Cicuta. *262,*
265 Hyp. *418.*

lower jaw immovable.
Theridion. *816.*

PARALYSIS:

Caust *222/3 227,* Acon. (Caust
222).

as result of dry cold winds.
Caust. *222.*

as result of suppression of
eruptions. Caust. *224.*

RHEUMATISM OF . . .
Caust. *227.*

SUNKEN CHEEKS.
Dros. *361,* Ver. alb. *853.*

STINGING.
Ant. crud. *55,* Caps. *202.*

EASY DISLOCATION OF JAW.
Rhus *711.*

EPITHELIOMA OF LIP AND
CHEEK.
Con. *323.*

TWITCHING MUSCLES.
Ant. tart. *66, 69.* Lyc. *517.*

Mez. *553.*

RHEUMATISM OF MAXILLARY
JOINTS.
Rhus. *711.*

GRACEFUL SPASMS AND
TWITCHINGS OF . . .
Stram. *779.*

SPASMS OF MUSCLES.
Bell. *122.*

NUMBNESS OF BONES OF NOSE
AND FACE AND CHIN.
Asaf. *103.*

CONVULSIVE MOVEMENTS.
Bell. *122.* Iod. *433.*

CRAMP IN FOREHEAD.
Asaf. *103.*

EXPRESSION OF GREAT FEAR
AND TERROR.
Acon. Stram. *774.*

DISTORTS FACE IN EFFORT TO
SPEAK.
Stram. *774.*

EXPRESSES FEAR, STUPIDITY.
Stram. *776.*

WITH ANXIOUS EXPRESSION.
Ver. alb. *853.*

FAINTING

AFTER SLEEP.
Carbo. v. *212.*

AFTER RISING.
Carvo. v. *212.* Opium. Phyt.
653

AFTER DEBILITATING LOSSES.
Carbo. v. *212.*

ON BELCHING.
Carbo. v. *212.*

FROM CRAVING FOR FOOD.
Sul. *791.*

ON STANDING A LONG TIME.
Nux. Mosch. *600.*

SUDDEN.
Sepia *743.*

WHILE KNEELING AT CHURCH.
Sepia. *743.*

FREQUENT DURING DAY.
Sul. *791.*

AFTER EVERY EXERTION.
Theridion. *817.*

ON SITTING UP.
Ver. vir. *860.*

FAINTNESS, SINKING ALL-GONE
FEELING.
Plumbum *669,* Sang. *731.*

FANTASIES.
See also MENTALS.

GETS IDEAS OF SUICIDE ON
SEEING BLOOD ON KNIFE.
Ars. Nat. sul. Thuja. Alum.
37.

THAT MIND AND BODY ARE
SEPARATED.
Anac. *49.*

THAT A STRANGER IS AT HIS
SIDE.
Anac. *49.*

THAT STRANGE FORMS
ACCOMPANY THEM.
Anac. *49.*

THAT HER HUSBAND IS NOT
HER HUSBAND.
Anac. *49.*

THAT HER CHILD IS NOT HER
CHILD.
Anac. *49.*

THINKS HIMSELF A DEMON.
Anac. *49.*

SCREAMS, AS IF TO CALL
SOMEONE.
Anac. *49.*

MANY DELUSIONS AND
ILLUSIONS.
Anac. *50.* Cann. *184.*

FEARS HE IS PURSUED.
Anac. *50.*

FEELS HE IS GOING TO HAVE A
FIT OR CREATE A SENSATION.
Arg. nit. *78.*

FEELS HE IS GOING TO JUMP OFF
A HIGH PLACE.
Arg. nit. *78.*

FEELS HE IS GOING TO DIE.
Cann. *184.*

FANCIES THIEVES ARE ABOUT.
Cann. *184.*

FANCIES MEN ARE BRIBED TO
KILL HIM.
Cann. *184.*

FEELS HE CAN FLY LIKE THE
BIRDS.
Cann. *184.*

FANCIES HE POSSESSES
INFINITIVE POWER OF VISION
& KNOWLEDGE.
Cann. *185.*

FANCIES HE POSSESSES
CREATIVE POWER, OR THE
WEALTH OF THE WORLD.
Cann. *185.*

FANCIES HE IS ON HORSEBACK,
IS SWIMMING, IS TRAVELLING
ETC.
Cann. *185*.

FANCIES HE HEARS MUSIC.
Cann. *187*.

HAS THE ILLUSION OF BEING A
PUMP, AN INKSTAND, A SAW,
SODA WATER,
HIPPOPOTAMUS, GIRAFFE,
FERN, TIN CAN — ALL
EXAGGERATED.
Cann. *185*.

HAS ILLUSION OF HEARING THE
NOISE OF COLOURS.
Cann. *187*.

FATIGUE
GREAT.
< talking. Alum. *38*.

MENTALLY AND PHYSICALLY.
Arn. *87*.

INDESCRIBABLE.
Caust. *223*.

ACID MUSCLE CONDITIONS FROM
FATIGUE.
Arn. Ferr. phos. *377*.
from 'growing pains' Ferr.
phos. *377*.

CHRONIC.
Lyc. *521*.

FEARS
OF:
accidents. Iod. *433*.
anticipation. Arg. nit. Ars.
Carbo. v. Lyc. Med. Phos. ac.
Sil. Gels. *384*. Thuja. Lyc. *514*.
Mez. *556*. Sil. *759*. Arg. nit. *78*.
81. Gels. *382*.

anticipation, but well able to
cope when the time comes.
Lyc. *514*.

anticipation, in the pit of
stomach. Mez. *556*, Lyc. *516*.
Phos. *644*.

appearing in public. Carbo. v.
Sil. (Gels) *384*.

assassination. Plumbum. *670*.

bed. Acon. *4*.

being alone. Ars. Arg. nit.
Acon. *4*. Con. *328*. Psor. *676*.
Stram. *771*. Tarent. *801*. Puls.
686. Kali carb. *468*. Lyc. *514*.
Lil. tig. *509*.

being approached. Ars. (Acon
4) Arn. *85*.

being bitten. Hyos. *413*. *415*.

being eternally lost. Cann.
184.

being injured. Hyos. *413*. *415*.

of being loathsome in body.
Lac. can. *491*.

being touched. Arn. *85*.

being washed (in children)
Sul. *786*.

death. Cann. *179*, Camph.
174. Ant. crud. *57*. Acon. *4*.
Alum. *36* Apis. *74*. Arg. nit. *78*,
Arn. *85* Calc. *158*. Ars. *95*.
Psor *676*, Ver. alb. *853*. *855*.
Cimic. *270*. *273*. *277*. Cocc. *290*.
Coffea *300*. Con. *328*. Glon.
389. Phos. *644*. Kali carb. *468*.

Lac. can. *491*. Lyc. *514*. Med. *534*. Nitric ac. *586. 589*. Opium. *616*.

of death – therefore useless to take medicine. Ars. *95*.

impending death. Acon. Arg. nit. *78*. Calc. *155*.

examinations through inability to fix attention. Aeth. Arg. nit. *82*.

examinations. Arg. nit. Aeth. *17*. Gels. *382*.

everything and everybody. Anac. *50*. Calc. *155*. Kali br. *466* Lac. can. *491*.

dogs. Bell. (Acon *4*).

evil. Iod. *433*.

impending evil. Alum. *37*. Calc. *155*.

the future. Kali carb. *468*.

failure. Sil. *758*.

falling. Gels. *383*. Lac. can. *491*.

apoplexy. Apis *74*. Glon. *391*.

disease. Calc. *156*. Lac. can. *491*.

ghosts. Acon. *4*. Kali carb. *468*, Lyc. *514*. Tarent. *800*. Sepia. *747*. Ran. b. *701*.

heights. Arg. nit. *82*.

imaginary black dog. Bell. *119*.

insanity. Cann. *179*. Sepia *747*.

knives. Nux. v. *608*.

people. Lyc. *514*.

poverty. Bry. (Acon *4*).

poison. Lach. Rhus. Bell. Kali brom. Hyos. *411*. Rhus. *708*. *712*.

having been poisoned. Glon. *389. 393*.

medicine being poison. Hyos *412*.

objects seen in imagination. Stram. *769*.

responsibility. Ars. (Gels. *384*).

snakes. *Lac. can. 487 491*, Bell. (Lac. can. *491*).

spiders. Lac. can. *491*.

suicide. Caps. *205*.

losing reasons. Alum. *37*, Calc. *155*.

thunder. Phos. (Acon. *4*) Phos. *644*. Rhod. *705*.

impending danger. Arg. nit. Gels. Caust. *225*. Tarent. *798*.

water, (hydrophobia) Bell. *120*. Stram. Hyos. *412, 414*.

consumption. Calc. *156*.

downward motion. Borax. (Gels. *383*).

monsters, animals or insects not present. Tarent. *800*.

heart stopping. Vib. *865*.

doing something dreadful while choreic tremblings are on. Viscum. *868*.

unusual sounds. Borax. *136*.

going to sleep. Camph. *174*.

going crazy. Cimic. *275*. Kali br. *467*, Lil. tig. *508*. Psor. *676*. Puls. *686*.

going to sleep because of
increased pain. Lach. *493*..

**PEOPLE ARE TRYING TO POISON
HER.**
Lach. *494*.

RELIGIOUS MONOMANIA.
Lach. *499*.

to go to sleep in case he should
die. Lach. *497*.

**THAT HEART OR BREATHING
WOULD STOP.**
Lac. can. *491*.

OF DARKNESS.
Med. *530*. Acon. *4*. Calc. *155*.
Cann *180*. Caust. *222*. Puls.
686. Lyc. *514*. Stram. Phos.
Cann. San. *733*. Stram. *774*.
Stram. Bell. *120*.

OF SOLITUDE OR DARKNESS.
Stram. *770*.

NOT **AFRAID IN THE DARK.**
Lac. can. *491*.

WITH RESTLESSNESS.
Ars. *92*. Calc. *155*. Cimic. *277*.
Tarent *798*.

**NIGHT FEARS OF CHILDREN
WITH SCREAMING, MOANING,
GRINDING TEETH, DREAMS.**
Kali br. *466*. *467*.

FELT IN STOMACH.
Kali carb. *468*. Mez. *552*.

STAGEFRIGHT.
Gels. *382*.

CLAUSTROPHOBIA.
Arg. nit. *81*.

EFFECTS OF FRIGHT.
Opium. *615*. *616*. Glon. *393*.

Opium. Acon. *5*. Gels. *384*.
Acon. Op., Ver. alb. Ign. *426*.

TERRIFYING IMAGINATIONS.
Lac. can. *487*.

UNREASONING FEAR.
Acon. *4*. Calc. *155*.

INTANGIBLE.
Acon. *4*. Tarent *798*.

MENTAL OR PHYSICAL.
Acon. *4*.

VISIBLE ON FACE.
Acon. *4*. Lac. can. *491*.

FEELINGS
SENTIMENTAL.
Ant. crud. *52*.

AMATIVENESS.
Canth. *197*.

**IRRESISTIBLE DESIRE TO TALK
IN RHYME.**
Ant. crud. *52*.

**BAD EFFECTS OF DISAPPOINTED
AFFECTIONS.**
Nat. mur. Calc. phos. Ant.
crud. *52*.

PEEVISH.
Ant. crud. *53*.

SULKY.
Ant. crud. *53*.

LOATHING LIFE.
Ant. crud. *53*.

**CONTINUAL ECSTATIC LONGING
FOR SOMEONE.**
Ant. crud. *55*.

**SOUND OF BELLS MOVES HIM TO
TEARS.**
Ant. crud. *55*.

FEELING OF EMPTINESS IN THE
HEAD.
Ant. crud. *55*.

CHILD CANNOT BEAR TO BE
TOUCHED OR LOOKED AT.
Ant. crud. *56*.

CHILD WANTS TO BE CARRIED
AND SOOTHED.
Ant. crud. *57*.

CHILD SCREAMS AND SHOWS
TEMPER AT EVERY LITTLE
ATTENTION.
Cham. Ant. crud. *57*.

CHILD IRRITABLE ON WAKING.
Ant. tart. *61*.

DISSATISFIED WITH
EVERYTHING.
Aur. *106*.

FEET
COLD.
Acon. *10*. Ammon. carb. *42*.
Ant. crud. *56*. Calc. *154*.
Carbo v. *211/2*. Cistus. *286*.
Mez. *554*. San. *735,* Sil. *751*.
Nat. mur. *569*.

> COLD.
Puls. Ledum. *503*.

COLD, DAMP.
Calc. *163*.

ONE HOT, ONE COLD.
Lyc. Puls. *683*.

COLD, WITH HEAT IN THE
HEAD.
Ammon. carb. *42*. Sepia *743*.

RIGHT FOOT COLD, LEFT FOOT
NORMAL.
Lyc. *515. 519*.

AS IF IN COLD WATER UP TO
ANKLES.
Sepia *744*.

HOT, SWELLING.
Bry. *150*. Ledum. *506*.
> in cold water. Ledum. *506*.

THRUSTS FEET OUT OF BED.
Sul. Puls. Cham. *237*. Med.
531. Sul. *782. 790*. Puls. Med.
Cham. 241. Sang. *731*. Sanic.
733. 735.

BURNING CORROSIVE PAINS.
Ruta *721*. Sul. *782*.
< NIGHT.
Sul. *782*.

BURNING.
Sul. Calc. s. *172*. Sul. *790*.

SOLES — BURNING.
Sul. *782. 791*. Sul. Pet. *632*.
pain in . . . Alum. *38, Ant.
crud. 54,* Ledum. *504*.
feel as if asleep. Cocc. *292, 297*.
painful. Coloc. *319,* Ledum.
506. Med. *532*.

TOES:
ball of big toe swollen and
painful. Ledum. *506*. Rhus.
710.
cramp. Calc. *155*.
hurt exceedingly when
stubbed. Colch. *305*.
numbness of . . . Nat. mur.
574.
ingrowing toenails *Magnetis
Polus Australis* (Nitric ac. *587*).
pain in . . . Colch. *298, 309*.
Ledum. *504*.

pain in ball of left big toe.
Colch. *309.*

sore between the toes. Sil. *751.*

FEET FEEL LIKE LEAD.
Nat. mur. *574.*

PAIN, LIKE DISLOCATION IN
RIGHT FOOT.
Cycl. *351.*

FEET GO TO SLEEP
IMMEDIATELY AFTER
SETTLING DOWN.
Ant. tart. *69.*

PAIN IN HEELS.
Pet. Cycl. *351. Pet. 628.*

SPLINTER-LIKE STITCHES IN
HEEL.
Pet. *632.*

SOLES BURNING.
Cham. *241,* Sang. *731.*

SOLE BECOMES CONCAVE
THROUGH CONTRACTION OF
FLEXORS.
Ruta. *719.*

CORNS, SENSITIVE, SMART,
BURN.
Sal. ac. Ran. b. *702.*

CHAPS.
Hepar. *405.*

CHILBLAINS ON HEEL.
Pet. *632.*

BUNIONS.
Rhus. *710.*

FEET CONTRACTED.
Ruta *719.*

EMACIATED.
Caust *229.*

HEAVINESS IN.
Alum. *38,* Arn. *94*

RHEUMATISM OF . . .
Ledum. *505.*

PURPLE AND MOTTLED.
Ledum. *506.*

CHOREA LIKE TWITCHING.
Stram. *775.*

PITTING ON PRESSURE.
Ledum. *506.*

FIDGETY.
Zincum. (Phos. *643*).

NUMB.
Pyrogen *691.* Cocc. *293.*

BLOATED.
Ledum. *503.*

PURPLE.
Ledum. *503.*

CRAMPS IN . . .
Colch. *309.* San. *735.* Stram.
777.

FEEL HEAVY.
Colch. *309.*

SWOLLEN, RED, SHINY.
Colch. *302. 309.* Ledum. *504.*

WITH SORE AND RAW SPOTS.
Allium. *31.*

HEELS BECOME NUMB.
Alum. *39.*

HORNY PLACES IN SOLES.
Ant. crud. *54. 56. 57.*

GREAT SENSITIVENESS OF SOLES
WHEN WALKING.
Ant. crud. *54.*

NAILS GROWING OUT OF SHAPE.
Ant. crud. *57.*

WALKS WITH FEET TURNED
  INWARD.
  Cicuta. *264*.

ANKLES – SPRAINED.
  Arn. *86. 87*.
  inflamed. Abrot. *2*.

PAINFUL.
  Urtica (Colch. *303*). Ledum.
  503.

CARRION-LIKE SMELL.
  Sil. *754*.

SUPPRESSED SWEAT.
  Sil. *756, 758*.

ACRID CORROSIVE SWEATING.
  Iod. *434*.

SWEATY 'SMELLY'.
  Sil. (Hepar *401/2*) (Pet. *632*).
  Sil. *751*. San. *735*.

FELON

AN INFLAMED SORE, ABSCESS
  OR BOIL.
  Iris. *452*. Ferr. phos. *380*.

FEMALE SEX

AMENORRHEA.
  Sepia *742*. *Tub. 837*.

DYSMENHORRHOEA.
  Cimic *274*. Ver. vir. *861*.
  with haemorrhoids. Collin.
  311.
  with agonizing, cramping
  pains. Coloc. *Mag. phos* (CM)
  (Ferr. phos. *375*).
  where pains double person
  up. Coloc. Opium *613*. Mag.
  phos. *523*.

> heat. Coloc. Mag. phos.
  523.

< cold. Coloc. Mag. phos.
  523.

from vexation Coloc. (Mag.
  phos. *523*).

preceded by aching bones.
  Pyrogen. *693*.

neuralgic. Mag. phos. *526*.

membranous. Mag. phos. *525*.
  Borax. *135*. Cham. *240*.

> continued movement.
  Pyrogen. *693*.

spasmodic. Vibernum. *863/6*.

< downward motion. Borax.
  135. Guaiacum. Ustilago. Vib.
  863.

pains of. Caul. *220*.

discharge of blood. Cham.
  240, Ipec. *441*.

with convulsions. Collin. *310*.

METRITIS.
  Tereb. *812*.

METRORRHAGIA.
  Stram. *777*, Calc. *161*, Caul.
  219. Sepia *742*.
  with steady flow of bright red
  blood. Ipec. *441*.

GALACTORRHOEIA.
  Calc. *162*.

CRAMPS IN PELVIS.
  > menses. Vib. *866*.

MENSTRUAL COLIC.
  Cham. *240*.

INFLAMMATION OF VULVA AND
  VAGINA.
  Canth. *196*.

ESCAPE OF FLATUS FROM
VAGINA.
Brom. *139*.

BREASTS:
swollen and secretion of milk
in woman of 50. Asaf. *105*.
appearance of milk in non-
pregnant elderly women.
Asaf. *105*.
inflammation in . . . Bell. *125*.
inflammation < motion. Bry.
143.
heavy. Bry. *147*.
stony hard. Bry. *147*.
pale but hard. Bry. *147*.
hot and painful. Bry. *147*.
pain in R. breast, to shoulder.
Sang. *730*.
flattened. Nux. mosch. *600*.
mastitis. Arn. *91*. Lac. can.
489.

MENSTRUATION:
painful. Puls. Caul. Cimic.
Mag. phos. 526.
> from flow. Cimic. *271*.
Sepia, Lach. Zinc. (Cimic.
271).

LOCHIA, BLACKISH, LUMPY,
OFFENSIVE.
Kreos. *468*.

GONORRHEAL DISCHARGE.
Thuja *827*.

WOMB.
misplacement. Aesc. *14*.
enlargements and induration.
Aesc. *14*.

BEARING DOWN:
> standing. Bell. (Lil. tig.
511).
> lying. Puls. (Lil. tig. *511*).
as if everything were coming
out through vagina. Lil. tig.
510. *512*.
must cross legs to prevent
protrusion. Sepia. Lil. tig. *510*.
512.

FALSE LABOUR PAINS.
Vib. *863*. *865/6* Caul. *218*.

OVARIES — AND WOMB
SWOLLEN AND TENDER.
Nux. mosch. *598*.
right ovary painful. Plat. Pall.
626.
> on pressure. *Pall*. *626/7*.
oophoritis (ovaritis) Pall. *627*.

HAEMORRHAGES AFTER
MISCARRIAGE.
Nitric ac. *598*.

DISTRESS AFTER MISCARRIAGE.
Lil. tig. *510*.

LABOUR:
pains irregular, spasmodic.
Caul *216*.
premature, with spasmodic
pains. Caul. *217*.
uterine atony. Caul. *218*.
with exhaustion. Caul. *218*.
with painful bearing down
pains. Caul. *218*.
with deficient pains. Caul.
218.
pains press upward. Cham.
240.

rigidity of Os. Cham. *240*.

distressing after-pains. Cham. *240*, VIb. *863*.

rash of lying in. Cham. *240*.

labour facilitated. Viscum. *686*, Cimic. *274*. *276* (WHEN THE SYMPTOMS AGREE)

with fainting fits and cramps. Cimic. *276*.

soreness of parts after . . . Arn. *89*.

to prevent haemorrhages after . . . Arn. *89*.

MILK:

child refuses it. Cina. *281*.

retarded due to mammary cicatrices. Graph. *399*.

stringy. Kali bich. *459*.

to dry up. Lac. can. *491*.

MENOPAUSE FLUSHES.

Glon. *390*.

FEVERS

HECTIC.

Abrot. *2*. Calc. *163*. Ptelea *683*. Sang. *730*.

SHORT SHARP ATTACK.

Acon. *8*. Cup. ac. (Cup. *348*).

INFLAMMATORY.

Acon. *10*.

DIPHTHERIC.

Ail. *28*.

TYPHOID.

Ail. *28*. Pyrogen. Arn. Bapt. *114*. Pyrogen. *689*.

CATARRHAL.

Bapt. *114*.

BILIOUS AND ENTERIC.

Bapt. *114*.

GASTRIC.

Bapt. *114*. Carbo v. *213*.

DYSENTERIC.

Bapt. *114*.

PUERPERAL.

Bapt. *114*.

MALIGNANT PUERPERAL.

Ail. *28*.

CEREBRO-SPINAL.

Bapt. *112*. *114*. Crot. *336*. *338*. Cup. *343*. Pyrogen *695*. Sal. ac. *723*. Ver. vir. *861*.

SEPTIC.

Bapt. *114*. Echinacea. Rhus. Pyrogen. *694 695*. *688/9*.

VIOLENT WITH SPASMS, IN NEWBORN.

Camph. *176*.

ADYNAMIC.

Carbo v. *213*.

SLOW.

Rhus. *715*.

CONTINUOUS.

Stram. *271*. Hyos. (Bell. *120*).

REMITTENT.

Bell. (Stram. *771*).

VIOLENT, MODERATELY HOT.

Stram. (Hyos. *412*).

NOT VERY HIGH, BUT WITH INSANITY.

Hyos. *412*.

SIMPLE ACUTE.

Aconite. (Pyrogen *688*).

MALARIA AND AFRICAN FEVERS.

Tereb. *812*.

INTERMITTENT (AGUE).
Urtica *646/7* China *256, 260*
Cistus *285* Ign. *426*. Nat. mur.
570. Calc. *163*.

**ACUTE NOT CONTINUOUS
FEVERS.**
Bell. *119*.

HYPERPYREXIA.
Ver. vir. *861*.

AT NOON ESPECIALLY.
Stram. 779.

LOW ZYGOMATIC TYPES.
Ail. *28*.

SHORT SUDDEN ATTACKS.
Acon. *6*. (Ferr. phos. *377*).

WITH BLOOD POISONING.
NOT Acon. *8*. Ail. *28*.

AFTER AN ABORTION.
Puls. Bell. *125*.

**WITH ALTERNATE CHILLS AND
HEAT . . .**
Calc. *163*.

AFTER ABUSE OF QUININE.
Calc. *163*.

AFTER ABUSE OF ICE WATER.
Carbo. v. *213*.

AFTER EMOTIONS.
Caps. *200,* Cocc. *298*.

WITH:
drowsiness. Bapt. *114*.
loquacity. Tub. *836*.
anxiety. Tub. *836*.
rapidly oscillating
temperature. Ver. vir. *861*.
thirst. Acon. *6*. China. *250*.
NO thirst. Aeth. *19*. Apis. *73*.
intense restlessness. Pyrogen.
693.

fear of solitude and darkness.
Stram. *770*.
headaches. Nat. mur. *573*.
nausea. Ipec. *443*.
pains in the head. Ipec. *441*.
flushes of heat. Glon. *389*.
bruised feelings. Bapt. *114*.

< AT NIGHT.
Ant. crud. *57*.

RESULTS OF FITS OF ANGER.
Cocc. *298*.

**SWEATING ALTERNATING WITH
DRY HEAT.**
Apis. *75*.

**CHILL ALTERNATING WITH
HEAT.**
Cocc. *298*.
cold sweat during typhoids.
Psor. *673*.
covered with boiling sweats
during . . . Psor. *673*.

**WANTS TO UNCOVER DURING
FEVER.**
Hyos. *408*.

VERY HOT DRY . . .
Bell. (Hyos *412*).

MUSCULAR POWER AFFECTED.
Gels. *385*.

IDIOPATHIC PYREXIA.
Pyrogen. *689*.

**AILMENTS FOLLOWING SEPTIC
FEVERS.**
Pyrogen. *695*.

IN INTERMITTENT FEVERS.
CHILL STARTS:
in thigh and between
shoulders or over one scapula.
Rhus. *708*.

in small of back. Rhus. *708*.

running up spine. Rhus. *708*.

SCARLET FEVER.

(SCARLATINA).

Ail. *26/9*. Crot. *338*.

body red. Ammon. carb. *43*.

malignant. Ammon. carb. *43*. *45*.

with swollen throat. Ammon. carb. *43*. *45*.

redness like scarlatina. Bell. *123*.

specific for scarlet fever. *Bell. 125*.

cure and prophylactic. Bell. *125*.

with hot dry skin. Ferr. phos. *380*.

with pains alternating from side to side. Lac. can. *489*.

with blood poisoning. Mur. ac. *563*. *565*.

chronic cases following . . . Psor. *676*.

with restlessness. Rhus. *707*, *712*.

with stupor. Tereb. *812*.

FIBROMA
TUMOUR CONSISTING OF FIBROUS TISSUE.
Calc. s. *172*.

FIG WARTS
RELATIVELY SMALL OR DISFIGURING PROTRUBERANCES.
Thuja *820*. See SKIN.

FINGERS
CONTRACTION.
Aeth. *20*. Caust. *229*.

SPASMODICALLY OPEN WHILE HOLDING THINGS.
Apis (dislikes heat), Agar *22* (likes heat).

PANARITIUM.
Ammon. carb. *43*.

INFLAMED.
Ammon. carb. *43*.

PAIN:
cramping. Acon. *10,* Nat. phos. *577*.

deepseated periostal. Ammon. carb. *43*.

arthritic. Ant. crud. *54*.

pain and swelling < motion. Bry. *144*.

stitching pains < motion. Bry. *144*.

rheumatic. Caul. *218/220*. Caust. *229*. Ledum. *504*.

tickling, pricking. Ptelea. *680*.

burning. Sul. *782*.

CRAMPS IN . . .
Calc. *155*.

WARTS ON . . .
Caust. *229*.

PARALYSIS OF . . .
Mez. *554*.

SUBSULTUS (TWITCHING).
Mez. *556*.

NUMBNESS IN . . .
Nat. mur. *574*. Con. *329*.

PARONYCHIA.
Nitric ac. *592*.

FISSURED, EVERY WINTER.
Pet. *629.*

CRACKED IN ENDS OF FINGERS.
Pet. *630. 633.*

OFFENSIVE ULCERS ON TIPS
OF . . .
Pet. *632.*

BLUE BLISTERS ON . . .
Ran. b. *700.*

SWOLLEN.
Sil. *751.*

UNHEALTHY, RAGGED, NEVER
LOOK CLEAN.
Pet. *631.*

TIPS COLD.
Chel. *251.*

AS IF SPLINTER OF GLASS IN
FINGER.
Sil. Nitric ac. *593.*

COLD, ICY COLD, FINGER TIPS.
Ant. tart. *69.* Carbo v. *212.*
Mez. *554.* Nux mosch. *597.*
Ver. alb., *855.*

THUMBS — NEEDLE LIKE
PRICKS.
Staph. *764.*

JOINTS — TEARING PAIN.
Staph. *764.*

NAILS — CRUSHED.
Ant. crud. *56.*
blue. Chel. *251.*
thick, black. Graph. *400.*
rough and yellow. Sil. *753.*
purulent onychia – as result of
vaccinations. Thuja *825.*

FIRST AID

COLLAPSE.
Carbo. v. 208 (200 C) Kali carb.
(Carbo v. *208*).

DYING.
Carbo. v. *208.*

'AIR HUNGER'.
Carbo v. *208.*

'CORPSE REVIVER'.
Carbo v. 208.

STRAINS.
Rhus, Calc. Nux. v. (Staph.
767).

MECHANICAL INJURIES.
Arn. *88.*

BRUISES.
Arnica (Colch. *302*). (Ledum
503) Arn. Ham. Ledum. Sal.
ac. (Staph. 767).

INJURIES OF 'SOFT' PARTS.
Arn. (Hyp. *419*).

INJURIES OF NERVES.
Hypericum 419. (Symphitum
794).

BLOWS FROM BLUNT
INSTRUMENTS.
Symphitum 794

SPRAINS.
Arn. Bellis (Symphitum *793*).

BLACK EYES.
Ledum. 504.

OPEN LACERATIONS AND CUTS.
Calendula (Ledum. *503*).

COLD PALE, PARALYSED,
MOTTLED WOUNDS.
Ledum. *503.*

TO HEAL LIP OF WOUNDS.
Hypericum. *419. 420*
(Symphitum *794*).

CLEAN CUTS, AS IN AN OPERATION.
Staph. *761, 765, 767*.

'PUNCTURED' WOUNDS.
Ledum. (Hyp. *418*) Hyp. *419.*
420, 423. Hyp. (Symphitum
794). *Ledum 502*.

AILMENTS FROM PUNCTURED WOUNDS.
Ledum. *502*.

SHOOTING FROM WOUND UP NERVE OF ARM.
Hyp. *418*.

FOR PREVENTION OF SEPSIS.
Calendula (Symphitum *793*).

BURNS.
Urtica urens. (Symphitum *794*)
Urtica *843*.
painless. Picric ac. *655*.

FRACTURES.
Calc. phos. Symphitum
(Staph. *767*).
compound. Arn. *91*.

EFFECTS OF SHOCK, MENTAL OR PHYSICAL.
Arn. (Symphitum *793*).

EFFECTS OF OVER EXERTION, STRAIN.
Symphitum. *793*.

SPLINTERS.
Ledum. *503*. Abrot. *2*.

MOSQUITO BITES.
Ledum. *507*.

GNAT BITES.
Cantharis. (*200* C) (Urtica *848*)
Canth. *196*, Arn. *88, 90*.

BEESTINGS.
Urtica urens *849* Arn. *88. 90*.

WASP STINGS.
Arn. (Urtica *849*). Arn. *88. 90*.

FLATULENCE (wind)
UP (BELCHING).
Ant. crud. *53*. Arn. *89*. Asaf.
,02. 105. Ornithogalum
(Graph. *398*) Ign. *430, 432*.

> from . . . Ant. tart. *67*.

violent. Arg. nit. *80*. *Carbo. v.*
204.

bitter. Bry. *149*.

loud. Asaf. *105*.

before and after a meal. Nitric
ac. *591*.

of red pepper taste. Caps. *204*.

rancid taste in mouth after.
Asaf. *103*.

DOWN (FLATUS)
offensive. Arn. *89*. Sil. *753*.

fetid. Asaf. *102, 105*. *Carbo v.*
204. 209. 211.

smells like rotten eggs. Psor.
673. Sul. *788*.

much flatulence. Calc. p. *166*.
China. Lyc. *Carbo v. 208/9*.
Arg. nit. Lyc. *518*.

no relief from passing flatus.
Arg. nit. *79*, Cham. *240*.
China. *260*. Cocc. *296*.

up and down. Ant. crud. *53*.

< at night. Carbo v. *204*.

< lying down. Carbo v. *204*.

**COMPLAINTS FROM
'OBSTRUCTED' FLATUS.**
Carbo v. *204*.

FLATULENT COLIC.
Cocc. *293. 296*.

**ACCUMULATES IN
HYPOCHONDRIA.**
Cham. *240*.

**FLATUS DOWN WITH COPIOUS
SWEAT ALL OVER BODY.**
Kali bich. *460*.

> **EMPTY ERUCTATIONS.**
Lyc. *518*.

FLATUS ABUNDANT.
Nitric ac. *591*.

BLOATING:
upper abdomen. *Carbo v.*
(Lyc. *521*).
lower abdomen. *Lyc. 521*.
whole abdomen. *China.* (Lyc.
521).

DISTENDED TO BURSTING.
Arg. nit. *79, Carbo v. 211,*
Cham. *240,* China *260.* Colch.
Lyc. (*China 260*) Cocc *293, 296.*
Lyc. 514/5.

FLU
COUGH.
Ammon carb. *41*.

COUGH AFTER . . .
Ammon carb. *41*.

GASTRIC FLUS.
Bapt. 112. 114.

'GRIPPE'.
Ant. tart. *68*, Pyrogen. *692*.

AFTER EFFECTS OF . . .:
intellectual unable to start
work again. Lyc. *515*.
neurotics. Scutellaria (Lyc.
515).
longstanding weakness.
Abrot. *2*. China. (Lyc. *515*).

WITH:
great restlessness, requiring
constant movement. Pyrogen
695.
terrible occipital headache.
Gels *383*.
chills up and down the spine.
Gels. *382*.
heaviness in legs. Gels. *382*.
tired sensation. Caust. *228*.
Gels. *382*.
excessive prostration. Bapt.
114.
sore bruised pains. Bapt. *114*.
violent diarrhoeia and
vomiting. Bapt. *112*.
drowsiness, dull red face and
besotted condition. Bapt. *111*.
typhoid conditions. Bapt. *111*.

PROPHYLACTIC.
Gels. 383.

AT START OF OTHER AILMENTS.
Gels. *382*.

RAPID ONSET.
Bapt. *111*. Camph. *173*.

SLOW ONSET.
Gels. (Bapt. *111*).

FOREIGN BODIES

EXPULSION FROM TISSUES OF
  E.G. FISH BONES, NEEDLES,
  BONE SPLINTERS ETC.
  Sil. *756.*

FORMICATION

SENSATION LIKE THAT OF ANTS
  CREEPING ON THE SKIN.
  Phos. ac. *638.*

of lower limbs. Aeth. *20,*
Alum, *39.*

of gluteal muscles. Agar *25.*
see also SKIN.

FUNGUS HAEMATODES
Calc. *160.*

FURY
See TEMPER.

G

GALACTORRHEA
MILK TOO PROFUSE. See
FEMALE SEX.

GALL BLADDER, STONES.

AGONY OF . . .
  Bell *124.*

COLIC.
  Chel. *247.* Kali carb. *471,* Lyc.
  518.

GALLSTONES.
  Chel. *251.*

GANGRENE.

Abrot. *2.* Carbo v. *210.*
Camph. *175.*

TENDENCY TO . . .
  Ammon. carb. *42.* Canth.
  194/5.

> FROM HEAT.
  Ars. *98.*

< FROM HEAT.
  Secale. Ars. *98.*

WITH RED STREAKS
  FOLLOWING COURSE OF
  LYMPHATICS.
  Pyrogen. *697.*

FOLLOWING ERYTHEMA.
  Can. b. *701*

WITH FEVER AND DELIRIUM.
  Ran. b. *701.*

GASTRALGIA

PAINS IN THE STOMACH.
  Carbo v. *212.* Cham. *240,* Ars.
  94. 97. Cina. *282.* See also
  STOMACH.

GASTRITIS.

INFLAMMATION OF STOMACH.
  See STOMACH.

GENITALIA.

MALE COMPLAINTS:
  generally Ferr. (Cimic. *271*).

  terrible erections. Picric ac.
  657.

  priapism. Picric ac. *657.*

  satyriasis. Picric ac. *657.*

  coldness of genitals. Picric ac.
  657.

itching prepuce. Puls. *684*.

hydrocele. Rhod. *705*. In children. Rhod. Abrot. *3*.

testes and epididymis intensely painful to touch. Rhod. *705*.

testicles – pain in . . . Caust. *228*.

pain < on touch. Staph. *763*.

relaxed, hanging down. Sul. *789*.

penis and testes swollen, purple-red. Arn. *89*.

itching on scrotum. Cocc. *297*. Graph. *400*. Pet *629*.

glans penis itching. Sul. *789*.

red erosions on glans penis. Thuja. *828*.

orchitis. Arn. *91*. Rhod. *705*.

varicocele. Collin. *311*.

with extreme constipation. Collin. *311*.

prostate problems. Con. *324*. Thuja. *828*.

nocturnal seminal emissions. Ferr. *370*.

< from seminal emissions. Kali br. *466*. Merc. *543*. Phos. ac. *636*.

involuntary discharge of semen. Sul. *789*.

soreness and moisture between scrotum and thigh. Hepar *406*, Sul. *789*.

FEMALE COMPLAINTS
Cup. (Cimic *271*).

Aur. *110*, Ferr. *373* Kali bich. *458*.

vagina: – prolapsed. Ferr. *373*.

burning in . . . Sul. *789*.

itching of . . . Kreos *479*.

scirrhus of . . Kreos *479*.

acrid discharge from . . . Med. *531*.

violent itching between labia. Kreos. *479*.

polyps and fistula. Calc. *162*.

pruritis vulvae with haemorrhoids. Collin. *312*. Tarent. *802*.

ovaries – pain in region. Lil. tig. *512*.

swollen. Lil. tig. *512*.

neuralgia. Mag. phos. *525*.

inflamed, pulsating. Lach. *497*.

atrophy of . . . Iod. *434*.

inflamed. Plat. *662*.

tumours and cysts. Plat. *662*.

nerve pains in . . . Coloc. *314*.

vulva itching with pimples. Sul. *789*.

as if vulva were enlarged. Sepia. *743*.

labia swollen. Borax. *136*. Kreos. *479*.

INTENSELY SENSITIVE.
Plat. *659*.

VOLUPTUOUS CRAWLING IN . . .
Plat. *659*.

PAINFUL SENSITIVENESS IN . . .
Plat. *659*, Thuja. *819*.

SEXUAL EXCITEMENT ON
WAKING.
Puls. *684*.

EFFECTS OF ONANISM OR
SEXUAL EXCESSES.
Staph. *763*.

PAINFUL, AS RESULT OF FLOW
OR URINE OR FAECES.
Sul. *789*.

CONDYLOMATA AROUND
GENITALS AND ANUS.
Thuja, Nitric ac. *592*, Thuja
819, 829.

SWEAT OF EXTERNAL
GENITALIA.
Pet. *631*, Sul. *789*, Thuja *819*.

HERPES ON PERINEUM.
Pet. *633*.

COVERED WITH APHTHAE.
Borax. *134*.

ITCHING AND BURNING.
Calc. *161*.

PAINS:
burning. Caps. *203*, Kreos *481*,
484. Tereb *810*.
burning. > heat. Ars. *94*.
smarting. Caps. *203*. Kreos.
484.
irritation and ulcerative. Ign.
431.

URETHRA:
haemorrhage from . . . Ferr.
phos. *380*.
ropy discharges from . . . Kali
bich. *456*.

needle-like stitches. Nitric ac.
592.
ulcers in . . . Nitric ac. *592*.
discharge from . . . Nitric ac.
592, Thuja *824*.
itching. Sul. *798*.

ERUPTIONS ON:
small blebs. Pet. *631*.
large blebs. Rhus. (Pet. *631*).

WARTS.
Thuja (Caust. *225*) Thuja *819*.

STITCHING IN URETHRA WHEN
NOT URINATING.
Caps. *203*.

BURNING IN URETHRA.
Ferr. *372*. Merc. *543*.

ODOUR OF FISH BRINE.
Sanic. *735*.

GINGIVITIS
INFLAMMATION OF GUMS. See
TEETH.

GLABELLA
FRONTAL BONE JUST ABOVE
NOSE.
Camph. *176*.

GLANDS
SWELLING OF . . .
Carbo v. *213*, Cistus *287*, Iod.
433. Con. *321*. Dros. *359 Iod.*
436 Merc. *537* Ail. *28*, Brom.
140 Phyt. *650* Rhus. *712. 715*.

SWELLING OF, WITH
EMACIATION OF BODY.
Iod. *436*, Theridion. *817*.

SWELLING ABOUT EARS.
Mur. ac. *563*.

SWELLING AFTER BRUISING.
Con. *321*.

PAIN IN SWOLLEN GLANDS.
Cocc. *298*.

SWELLING OF:
parotid. Apis, Ammon. carb.
45, Cham. *240*, Kali bich. *456*,
Nitric ac *591*.

inguinal. Ars. *95*, Merc. *542*.
Nitric ac. *593*.

submaxillary. Calc. *160*, Dros.
Cham. *240*. Calc. *155*. Lac.
can. *490* Phyt. *650*. Nitric ac.
591, *593*. Rhus. *712*.

mesenteric. Calc. *161*. Iod.
434, 436.

lymphatics. Tarent. *799*.

neck glands. Tub. *833*, Calc.
162 Cistus *287/8* Graph. *400*.

cervicals. Calc. *162*, Con. *328*.
Dros. *358*, Iod. *434*.

axillary. Con. *329*. Crot. *333*.

lymphatic glands of abdomen.
Iod. *436*. Nat. phos. *577*.

hypertrophy of all glands
other than mammary. Iod.
434, 436.

glands in groin (buboes)
Hepar *405*.

ABSCESSES OF INGUINAL
GLANDS.
Hepar. *405*.

PAIN IN CERVICAL GLANDS.
Ign. *430*.

ADENOMATEOUS
(OVERGROWTH OR TUMOUR)
OF GLANDS.
Dros. *359*.

MALIGNANT, CANCEROUS.
Con. *321*.

STONY, HARD.
Con. *321*, Iod. *433* Brom. *140/
2*, Calc. *155*, Ail. *27* Ammon.
carb. *45*.

TORPID SWELLINGS.
Calc. s. *172*.

INFLAMMATION AND
INDURATION.
Calc. *164*. Cistus. *287*.

SUPPURATING AND
INDURATING.
Ars. *97*.

SUPPURATIONS, SUDDEN AND
RAPID.
Hepar *402*.

slow and slow to heal. Sil.
(Hepar *402*).

SELDOM SUPPURATING.
Brom. *140*.

STITCHING PAINS.
< movement. Bry. *144*.

< FROM TAKING COLD.
Con. *321*.

MESENTERIC ATROPHY.
Calc. *161*. Drops. *358*.

THYROID:
enlargement and hardness.
Brom. *140*, Iod. *434, 436*.

constrictive pain round . . .
Crot. casc. (Crot. *339*).

acute pain in . . . Iod. *434*.

tender and enlarged. Ail. *28*.

GLIOMA OF BRAIN
(TUMOUR).
Bell. *118*.

GLOSSOPLAGIA
PARALYSIS OF THE TONGUE.
Caust. *229*.

GLOTTIS
Bell. *124*, Brom. *138*.

GOITRE
Ammon. carb. *42*, Brom. *140*.
Cistus *285*, *287*, Iod. *433*.

WITH FAMILY T.B. HISTORY.
Dros *359*, Tub. bov. (Dros.
359).

BASEDOW'S DISEASE.
Ferr. *370*.

BASEDOW'S DISEASE AS RESULT
OF SUPPRESSION OF MENSES.
Ferr. *370*.

EXOPHTHALMIC GOITRE.
Ferr. *374*, Iod. *436* (but only if
Iodine symptoms too)

IF WITH 'IGNATIA MENTAL
SYMPTOMS'.
Ign. *429* (or use 'Chronic –
Sepia (Ign. *429*).

HARD.
Iod. *434*. Nat. phos. *577*.

GONAGRA
GOUT OF KNEE JOINT. See
KNEES. and GOUT.

GONORRHEA.
Calc. *166*, Thuja, Nat. sul.
582. Thuja *819*.

WHITE DISCHARGE.
Caps. *201*.

EXCESSIVE SENSIBILITY OF
PARTS.
Caps. *201*.

LATER STAGES OF . . .
Caps. *203*.

YELLOW DISCHARGE.
Puls. Kali sul. *475*.

ACUTE.
Thuja. Nitric ac. Med. *528*.

ACUTE AND CHRONIC.
Thuja. 828.
alternatively use Thuja and
Nitric acid (Nitric ac. *589*).

GOUT
Abrot. *2. Colch. 302.*

PAIN UNBEARABLE.
Cham. Colch. *305*, Ledum.
503.

RHEUMATIC.
Rhus. *710*.

FEET RED, SWOLLEN, VERY
PAINFUL.
Urtica. *848*.

STIFF JOINTS.
Caps. *205*.

WITH STIFF FINGERS.
Agar. *25*.

GONAGRA.
Caust. *229*.

CHRONIC.
Kali carb. *472* (low potencies)

BEGINNING IN LOWER LIMBS
AND ASCENDING.
Ledum. *507*.

WITH FEAR OF BEING
APPROACHED.
Arn. *88*.

WHERE NODULES BECOME
PAINLESS.
Ant. crud. *58*.

METASTISING TO HEART OR
STOMACH.
Colch. *303*.

WITH PASSING OF GRAVEL
(URATES).
Urtica. *847*.

IN PERSONS OF VIGOROUS
CONSTITUTION.
Colch. *308*.

< SLIGHTEST MOVEMENT.
Colch. *305*.

< COLD DAMP WEATHER.
Colch. *305*.

> COLD.
Ledum. *504*.

GRIPPE
(FLU) See FLU

H

HAEMATEMESIS
VOMITING OF BLOOD. See
VOMITING.

HAEMATURIA
ANY CONDITION IN WHICH THE
URINE CONTAINS BLOOD.
Arn. *89*, Ars. *93*. Kreos. *483*.
Tereb. *812*.

HAEMOPTYSIS
SPITTING OF BLOOD.

HAEMORRHAGES
GENERAL HAEMORRHAGIC
DIATHESIS.
Ferr. *371*, Kreos *482/3*
Millifolium (Hyp. *417*).

FROM ALL OUTLETS.
Crot. Sul. ac. Ferr. China *260*
Crot 335. Ferr. phos *379*. Ipec.
446, Tereb. *813*.

WITH BRIGHT BLOOD
(ARTERIAL) FROM ANY
OUTLET.
Ferr. phos *379*, Ipec *446*.

PROFUSE.
Phos. Kreos. *482/3*. Nitric ac.
593.

WITH FLOWING BLOOD,
DIFFICULT TO COAGULATE.
Phos. *646*.

COMING IN GUSHES.
Ipec. *446*, Lac. can. *488*.

EASY BLEEDING.
Phos. *643*.

EASY BLEEDING, WITH FEAR OF
DEATH.
Acon. *5*. Ars. *95*.

CLOTS EASILY.
Lac. can. *487*.

DO NOT CLOT EASILY.
Ipec. (Lac. can. *487*).

PASSIVE.
Phos. ac. *639*.

IN FIRST STAGES ONLY.
Ferr. phos. *379*.

IN PALE ANAEMIC PEOPLE.
Ferr. phos. *379*.

POST PARTEM.
Secale, Ipec. *443*, Nitric ac. *593*.

WITH YELLOW SKIN.
Crot. *337*.

CEREBRAL.
Arn. *86*, Opium. *612*.

WITH FLOW OF URINE.
Alum. *36*.

DARK.
Ammon. carb. *44*, China. *260*, Crot. *335*.

DRAWS OUT INTO LONG BLACK STRINGS.
Crocus (Kali bich. *453*).

OF:
nose. Sal. ac. *726*, Crot. *335*.
stomach. Cal. ac. *726*
gums. Sal. ac. *726*.
arms. Tereb. *810*.
bowels. Tereb. *810* Alum. *36*. Nitric ac. *593*.
lungs. Tereb. *812*.
uterus (hot) Bell. *125*, Caul. *220*, Ipec. *446*.
uterus, with internal trembling. Caul. *220*.

WITH:
great prostration. Crot. *335*.

shaking chill. China *260*.
faintness. China *260*.
loss of sight. China *260*.
ringing in ears. China *260*.
weakness. China. Ferr. *373*, China (Ipec. *446*).

AFTER MISCARRIAGE.
Nitric ac. *593*.

FROM OVER-EXERTION.
Nitric ac. *593*.

AS RESULT OF TEMPER.
Cham. *237*.

AFTER MECHANICAL DAMAGE.
Arn. *89*.

HAEMORRHOIDS.
See PILES.

HAEMORRHOPHILIA
TENDENCY TO BLEEDING PILES.
Ferr. *371*.

HAIR
FALLING OUT.
Ant. crud. *52*, Carbo v. *210*, Ail. *29*, Nitric ac. *590*. Sepia *740* Graph. *398* Lyc. *516*. Med. *530*.

ITCHING ON HEAD.
Ant. crud. *52*.

TANGLING AT TIPS.
Borax *132, 136*.

STICKING TOGETHER.
Borax. *136*.

BALDNESS.
Abrot. *2*.

BECOMES GREY TOO SOON.
Lyc. *516*.

WHITE PATCH OF HAIR
NORMALISED.
Psor. *672*.

DRY, LUSTRELESS, ROUGH
HEAD OF HAIR
Psor. *673*.

COARSE, LUSTRELESS,
UNKEMPT.
Sul. *786*.

GROWTH OF HAIR ON PARTS
OTHERWISE NOT COVERED
BY HAIR.
Thuja. *829*.

HALOGENS
Brom. *138* (Chlorine, Iodum.
435).

HANDS
CRACKED.
Pet. 628. Sanic. *735*.

< COLD WEATHER.
Pet. *629*.

SHAKING.
Mag. phos. *525*.

ITCHING.
Mur. ac. *565*.

TWITCHING.
Opium. *613*.

SWELLING.
Colch. *309*.

NUMBNESS.
Glon. *388,* Cocc. *292, 296*. Nat.
mur *574*. Pyrogen *691*

FEEL SWOLLEN.
Cocc. *292*.

DEFORMED.
Caust. Med. (Caul. *220*).

ITCHING ERUPTION ON . . .
Carbo v. *213*.

FLABBY, 'BONELESS'.
Calc. *154*.

TREMBLING.
Agar. *24,* Allium *30,* Ant. tart.
68. Merc. v. *545*. Merc. *538*
543. Ledum *505,* Cocc. *297*.
Sul. *790*.

BURNING.
Phos. *643*. Sang. *731*. Sul. *782*.
790.

BURNING ITCHING, HOT
SWOLLEN RED.
Agar *24*.

BURNING, SPREADING OVER
BODY.
Chel. *251*.

BURNING ERUPTIONS.
Cicuta *263*.

RHEUMATOID ARTHRITIS IN . . .
Caul. *220*.

RHEUMATOID ARTHRITIS, < IN
THUNDERSTORMS.
Rhod. (Caul *220*).

HANDS 'FALL ASLEEP' AT
NIGHT.
Sil. *753*.

FIRST ONE HAND, THEN THE
OTHER GOES TO SLEEP.
Cocc. *292*.

FIRST HANDS, THEN FEET GO TO
SLEEP ALTERNATELY.
Cocc. *297*.

ALTERNATELY HOT AND COLD.
Cocc. *296*.

VIOLENT DRAWING PAINS IN
RIGHT THUMB.
  Coloc. *319*.
'CHAPS'.
  Hepar *405*, Pet. *629*.
ONE HAND HOT, ONE COLD.
  Puls. *683*.
HANDS HOT WITH FEET COLD,
OR HANDS COLD WITH FEET
HOT.
  Sepia *748*.
CHOREA-LIKE TWITCHING.
  Stram. *775*.
CRAMPS IN . . .
  Stram. *777*.
CRACKS ON BACK OF . . .
  Pet. *630*.
TISSUE HARDENS.
  Pet. *631*.
RAW FROM WRISTS TO FINGERS
WITH CONSTANT WATERY
OOZING.
  Pet. *632*.
TREMBLING, WITH FLUSHES OF
HEAT OVER WHOLE BODY.
  Plat. *661*.
ALWAYS SEEM TO HAVE DIRTY
HANDS.
  Psor. $\overline{673}$.
COLD AND CLAMMY.
  Pyrogen. *691*.
BLISTER-LIKE ERUPTIONS.
  Ran. b. *700*.

HAYFEVER
  Psor. 672.
SENSITIVE TO ODOUR OF
FLOWERS.
  Allium *30*, Sang. *731*.

SENSITIVE TO ODOUR OF PEACH
SKINS.
  Allium *30*.
WITH EYES SMARTING.
  Ran. b. *699*.
WITH NOSE STUFFED.
  Ran. b. *699*.

HEAD
PAIN:
  rheumatic. Caust. *226*.
  as if head were numb and
  pithy. Graph. *398*.
  painful to touch. Merc. *541*,
  Mez. *551*.
  burning. Ars. *94*. Canth. *195*,
  Sul. *783*.
  pressive in forehead. Asaf.
  102. Mez. *553*.
  of fractured skull. Glon. Bell.
  117.
  pains < motion. Bry. *143*,
  Calc. p. *167*.
  bursting. Caps. *199, 200*.
  from occiput, over top of
  head, running down over
  right eye. Sang. *730*.
  over left eye. Spig. (Sang.
  730).
  INside head. Stram. *778*.
  nocturnal throbbing pain in
  and around . . . Asaf. *102*.
FEELS:
  too large. Arn. *88*. Chel. *249*.
  Caps. *202, 205*. Cimic *272/3*
  Glon. *388*. Nux. mosch. *598*.
  heavy as lead. Carbo v. *212*.
  Pet. *633*.

hollow. Cocc. *298*.

as if empty space were between brain & cranial bones. Caust. *222*.

'bound'. Cycl. *351*. Nitric ac. *590*.

as if in a vice. Merc. *544*, Nitric ac. *590*.

as if head were separated from body. Psor. *672*.

as if there were not enough room for the brain. Psor. *672*.

as if wind went through the head. Sanic. *733*.

UNABLE TO HOLD HEAD UP.
Calc. p. *167*, Nat. mur. Abrot. Sanic *735*.

INCLINES HEAD FORWARD TO EASE PAIN.
Sanic. *735*.

TOO WEAK TO LIFT HIS HEAD OFF THE PILLOW.
Colch. *303*.

SPASMODIC DRAWING OF HEAD BACKWARDS.
Cicuta *263*.

RETRACTED OR BENT FORWARD AND STIFF.
Cicuta *264*.

ERUPTIONS ON VERTEX.
Graph. *398*.

SENSATION:
as if brain moved. Ars. *100*, Cycl. *351*, Sul. *785*.

as if cord tied tightly round brain. Asaf. *101*. Sul. *785*.

as if brain were pressed against skull. Calc. p. *167*, Glon. *388*.

of nail being driven into brain. Asaf. *102*.

as if bolt driven from neck to vertex. Cimic. *275*.

of skull being soft and thin. Calc. p. *167*.

of opening and shutting of parietal region. Vib. *865* and of occipital region. Cocc. (Vib. *865*).

that head will burst. Bell. *119*, Cimic. *273*.

< ascending. Cimic. *273*.

swishing and gurgling. Asaf. *102*.

HOT.
Bell. *123*, Calc. p. *167*. Camph. *176*. Cocc. *296*, Ferr. *372*.

HOT, WITH COLD FEET.
Ferr. *372*.

VERY SENSITIVE TO COLD.
Bell. *117*.

COMPLAINTS FROM GETTING THE HEAD COLD.
Bell. *117*.

SWEATY.
Calc. Sil. Calc. p. *165*.

COLD HEAD.
Calc. *154*, Calc. p. *167*.

PROFUSE SWEAT ON HEAD.
Calc. 156.

HUMID BURNING ERUPTIONS ON TOP OF . . .
Sul. *787*.

VERY HOT.
Stram. *775*.

CEREBRAL CONGESTION.
Ver. vir. *860*.

SORE TO TOUCH.
Sil. *752*.

WITH ITCHING ON FOREHEAD.
Sul. *787*.

FRACTURES OF SKULL.
Arn. *88*.

SCALP:
itching. Graph *398*, Merc. *541*.
Mez. *553*. Puls. *683*.

scabs on. Mez . . . *553*.

crawling in . . . Ran. b. *700*.

dandruff on . . . Thuja *828*.
Nat. mur *573*.

inflamed pimples on hairy . . .
Sul. *787*.

temple and scalp alive with
irrepressible pulsations. Sang.
729.

heat on crown of . . . Sul. *787*.

RUSH OF BLOOD TO HEAD.
Bell. Glon. Ferr. phos. *380*.

DIZZY, WITH BLURRED VISION.
Gels. *385*.

FULLNESS AT BACK OF HEAD
AND NECK.
Gels *385*.

HYPERAEMIA OF BRAIN.
Glon. *390*.

NAUSEA FELT IN HEAD.
Cocc. *299*.

OLD JARS TO HEAD
Glon. *390*.

ROLLING FROM SIDE TO SIDE.
Pyrogen *691*.

HOT FEELING ON TOP.
Nat. sul. *584*.

RHYTHMICAL PRESSURE IN
HEAD.
Ruta. *720*.

STITCHES IN LEFT FRONTAL
BONE, ONLY FROM READING.
Ruta *720*.

AFTER-EFFECTS OF INJURIES TO
HEAD OR CONCUSSION.
mental. Nat. sul. *582*. *584*.

neuralgic. Arn. (Nat. sul. *582*)
Arn. *88*.

TENSION, WITH NAUSEA.
Nitric ac. *590*.

TWITCHING.
Opium. *613*.

AS IF CONSTRICTED.
Graph. *398*, Merc. *541*, Sul.
Nitric ac. *593*.

CARIES OF BONE.
Mez. *551*.

COMPRESSION OF THE BRAIN.
Asaf. *101*.

NUMBNESS OF . . .
Cham. Plat. Asaf. *105*.

FONTANELLES SLOW TO CLOSE.
Calc. 153, 156. 159. Calc. p.
165, 167, 170

PAINS RELIEVED BY PASSING
FLATUS.
Carbo v. *208*.

CONSTRICTIONS IN
CEREBELLUM.
Camph. *176*.

CRUSTS ON HEAD OF INFANT.
Calc. *162*.

SCRATCHES HEAD ON WAKING.
Calc. *156*.

HEADACHES
PAIN:

throbbing. Glon. Bell. *117, 124*
Cham. *218*. Crot. *338*. Colch.
302 Ign. *430*. Iris. *450*. Glon.
388/9. Lyc. *516*. Mag. phos *527*
Camph. *176*. Canth. *195*.
Caps. *200*. Glon. *388*. Picric
ac. *656*.

left side. Acon. *9*. Caps *200*.

behind forwards. Bell. *121*.

violent. Caust. *224,* Mez. *551*.
Sil. *750*. Phos ac. *637*.

intolerable. Acon. *9*. Chel.
249. Glon. *394*.

severe. Ail. *26/7*. Bell *121*. Bry.
147.

acute – NOT Nat. mur. Bry.
147.

chronic. Nat. mur. (Bry. *147*).
Ammon. carb. *41*. Nat. mur.
574. Phos ac. *637*.

cutting. Lach. *499,* Sang. *729*.

congestible. Glon. Bell. *117*.
Cham. *238*. Cocc *293*. Crot.
336. Merc. *541*.

tearing. Calc. *159*. Caps. *200*.

shooting. Caps. *200,* Cimic.
275.

shooting. < at rest. Caps. *200*.
Cicuta *261*.

pressing. Caps. *200*. Carbo v.
212.

burning. Acon. *9*. Kali bich.
459.

stabbing. Alum. *37*. Cham.
239.

hammering. Ammon carb. *41*.
Ferr. *370/1*. Lach. *497*. Nat.
mur. *570*.

migraine type. Cann *179*

paroxysmal. Sang. *729*.

'deep in'. Tub. *833*. *835*.

periodical. Tub. *837*.

intermittent. Nitric ac. *592*.

intense pain, as of needles.
Tarent. *801*.

in or behind the eyes.
Theridion. *815*.

occipital. Stram. *772*. Tarent.
801. Bac. (Tub. *834*). Bry. *148*.
Caps. *202*. Carbo v. *210*. *212*.
Murex *565*. Nux v. *603* Nux
mosch. *596*. Nat. phos. *576*.
cocc. *292/3 299*. Chel *249* Crot.
338. Gels. *383*. Pet. *629*. *631*.
Phos ac. *637*.

starts in occiput. Calc. *159*.
Cimic. *275*. Lach. *499,* Sang.
729. Sil. *752*.

in sinciput and then in
occiput. Cina *282*, Coloc. *318*,
Lil. tig. *512*.

frontal. < stooping. Bry. *148*.
Ign. *430*.

frontal. Staph. *762*. Theridion.
815. Vib. *864*. Nat. phos. *576*.
Bry. *148*. Caps. *200, 202*.
Cicuta *261*. Ferr. phos *379*.

in vertex. Cimic. *272*. Ferr.
371. Lach. *499*. Ver. alb. *853*.

occiput, alternately opens and shuts. Cocc. *299*.

vertex, alternately opens and shuts. Cann. (Cocc. *299*).

IN NAPE OF NECK (AS IF ALTERNATELY OPENING AND CLOSING).
Cocc. *293*.

SYPHILITIC.
Thuja. *828*.

SYCOTIC.
Thuja *828*.

IN BONES OF SKULL.
Ipec . . . Ptelea. *680*.

SICK HEADACHES:
due to over-exposure to sun. Glon. Nat. mur. Phos. Spig. Stann. Sang. *728*.

starts in morning. Stann. *728*.

grows more intense during the day. Stann. *728*.

< towards evening. Stann. *728*.

with nausea and vomiting. *Sang. 730*.

< FROM:
being touched. Staph. *765*.

wet cold weather. Rhod. *704*.

eating. Nux v. *603*.

standing Ran. b. *698*.

heat. Phos. *641*.

stooping forward. Agar. Aesc. *12*, Ign. *430*

motion. Anac. *48*, Bell. *121*. *Bry. 143*. Cimic. *272*. Cocc. *294*. Glon. *394*. Stram. *772*. Theridion. *815*.

pressure. Bell. *121*. Cicuta *262*.

in open air. Cina *282*, Coffea *300*, Glon. *390*. Iris. *450*.

on rising in the morning. Cycl. *349*. Lyc. *516*. Nux. v. *603*. Sang. *729*.

shaking head. Glon. *389*. *390*.

on damp rainy days. Glon. *388*.

after mental exertion. Glon. *388*.

in evening. Iris. *450*.

coughing. Iris. *450*.

walking. Agar. Aesc. Bell. *121*. Caps. *200*. Cina *282*.

bending head backwards. Bell. (Glon. *394*).

moving eyes. Nux. v. *603*.

lying. Glon. *394*. Ran. b. *698*, Stram. *772*, Theridion *815*.

with head low. Glon. *394*.

wine. Glon. *394*, Rhod. *704*.

jar. Stram. *772*.

change of position. Crot. *338*.

9 a.m. Kali carb. *471*.

FROM:
binding something round head. Arg. nit. *80*. Bell. Mag. phos. *527*.

standing. Iris. *450*.

washing. Psor. *676*.

bending head backwards. Bell. (Glon *394*).

covering head. Glon. *394*, Sil. *750*.

UNcovering head. Bell.
(Glon. *394*).

pressure. Ammon carb. *43*,
Bell. *121*. Bry. *145*, Glon. *394*,
Pall. *627*.

after eating Anac. *48*. Sepia
740.

motion. Caps. *200*, Iris, *450*.

lying down. Sang. *729*.

sleep. Sang. *729*.

cold air. Ars. Phos. Ledum.
503. Phos. *641*.

walking. Ran . . . b. *698*.

nosebleed. Psor. *676*.

NERVOUS HEADACHES.
Asaf. *102*. Gels. *383*. Thuja
828. Tub. *837*. Anac. *48*.

SICK HEADACHES.
Iris. *450*, Nat. mur. *574*.

BEGINNING WITH BLUR BEFORE
EYES.
Iris. *450* Anac. *48*, Crot. *338*,
Ipec. *444*. Iris *451*, Collin. *311*,
Ptelea. *679*.

AFTER A MEAL.
Ammon carb. *42*.

AFTER UTERINE
HAEMORRHAGES.
Glon. *389*.

AFTER FALL ON OCCIPUT.
Hyp. *422*.

AFTER ALCOHOLIC DRINKS.
Ant. crud. *53*.

AFTER BATHING.
Ant. crud. *53*.

AFTER TEMPORARY BLINDNESS.
Kali bich. *456*. *459*.

BEFORE TEMPORARY
BLINDNESS.
Sil. (Kali bich. *456*).

OF DRUNKARDS.
Agar. *25*, Nux. v. *603*.

PAIN:
temporal. Phos. ac. *637*, Glon.
388, *Lyc. 516*. Ran. b. *698*.
Staph. *762*, Thuja *819*.
Bacillinum. (Tub *834*).

pressing inwards and
outwards. Staph. *765*.

shooting from frontal to
temporal bone. Ruta *720*.

shooting from temporal to
occiput. Ruta *720*.

'blinding' headache. Caust.
Kali bich. *456*. Thuja *826*.

pulsating. Lach. *497*.

from root of nose into
forehead. Mez. *552*.

constant. Nat. sul. *585*.

hemicrania. Cham. *239*.

violent stitches in brain.
Alum. *37*. Cham. *239*.

AS IF:
bruised brain, with nausea.
Ipec. *444*.

head were nailed up. Acon. *9*.
Thuja, Coffea *300*, Thuja *819*.
head would burst. Ant. crud.
55, Bry. *145*, Calc. *159*, Glon.
388/90 394. Crot. *338*. Lach.
497, 499. Cocc. *295*. Con. *327*.
Kali bich. *489*. Nat mur. *572/3*,
Nux mosch. *597*. Nux. v. *604*.
Ver. vir. *862*. Sang. *729*, Sepia
743, Sul. *784*. Sil. *750*. *752*.

bound with tight hoop of iron.
Tub. *839*.

head were distended from
within outwards. Arn. *86*,
Ferr. *371*

head were hollow. Cocc. *295*.

eyes would be torn out. Cocc.
296.

stabbed with a knife. Alum.
37. Bell. *121*.

head were enlarged. Plat. *662*.

hair pulled. Alum. *37*.

WITH:

diarrhoeia in school girls.
Calc. p. *166*.

fullness and heaviness Acon.
9. Amil nit. Glon. *391*.

vertigo. Acon. *9*. Chel. *249*.
Cocc. *295*. Collin. *311*. Iris.
451.

shaking head. Acon. *9*. Ferr.
370.

nausea. Bell. *121*, Chel. *249*.
Cocc. *294*. *296*. Sepia *740*.
Sang. *729*. Nux. v. *603*. Ferr.
370. Ipec. *443/4*. Iris. *451*. Nat.
phos. *574*. Theridion. *815*.

flickering before eyes. Cycl.
349.

back of head cold. Sil. *750*.

red face. Bell. (Crot. *332*).
Ferr. phos. *380*.

aversion to eating or drinking.
Ferr. *370*, Sepia *740*.

soreness. Ferr. phos. *380*.

vomiting. Ferr. phos. *380*.

dimness of vision. Gels. *383*.

red hot eyes. Glon. *389*.

sense of fullness in head.
Glon. *391*.

violent pains over eye. Iris.
451, Theridion. *815*.

facial neuralgia. Iris. *451*.

salivation. Nat. sul. *580*.

bloated stomach, Lyc. Kali
bich. *456*.

blotched, bloated, pimply
face. Kali bich. *456*.

sallow, yellow face. Kali bich.
456.

FROM:

walking in the sun. Stram.
772.

deranged stomach. Ant. crud.
53.

a cold. Ant. crud. *53*.

suppressed emotions. Ant.
crud. *53*. Cimic. *275*. Caps.
205.

sunrise to sunset. < midday.
Nat. mur. *574*.

AS RESULT OF:

vaccination. Thuja. *822 824/7*.

sunstroke. Glon. *390*,
Theridion. *815*, Gels. Bell.
Ver. vir. *860*.

(for after-effects of sunstroke)
Glon. *392*, Sang. *728*.

overwork. Picric ac. *656*.

SENSATION OF LUMP OF ICE IN
VERTEX.
Ver. alb. *853*. *856*.

WITH INABILITY TO URINATE.
Con. *327/9*.

WITH A COUGH.
Caps. *203*, Lyc. *516*.

PULSE HIGH, OUT OF PROPORTION TO TEMPERATURE.
Picric ac. *656*.

IN SMALL SPOTS.
Kali bich *453. 455*.

KNEES GIVE WAY DURING HEADACHE.
Glon. *390*.

WITH INFLAMMATION OF BRAIN.
Bell. Glon. *394*.

HEART

PAINS:
stitching. Agar. *23*, Anac. *49*.

stitching, < movement. Bry. *144*.

pressing pains in cardiac region. Asaf. *101* Cann. *183*.

cutting and stinging. Colch. *305, 309*.

burning pains round heart. Ars. *94*.

dull . . . Crot. *337*.

constriction around heart. Asaf. *103*.

cardiac attacks. Ammon. carb. *44*, Cimic. *273*.

clutching and crampy. Vib. *865*, Theridion. *817*.

ANGINA:
Ammon carb. *43*, Mag. phos. *525*. Tarent. *802*.

violent attacks. Arn. *88* (Aur. *107*) Spig. (Gels. *384*).

with violent beating of heart. Aur. *107. 110*. Tarent *802*.

pain in chest and down left arm. Cimic. *273*, Tarent *802*.

symptoms of . . . Cimic. *274*.

intercurrent remedy with Aurum . . . Glon. *390*.

heart cramp. Vib. *864*.

PULSE:
intermittent. Kali carb. *471*. Mur. ac. *564*, Nat. mur. *570. 573*

irregular. Aur. *109* . . . Gels. *384. 386*. Kali carb. *471*. Nat. mur. *570*.

violent beating. Aur. *110*.

fast. Acon. *10*. Ars. *99*. Collin. *312*. Pyrogen *692. 695*.

feeble circulation. Carbo v. *207*.

weak and irregular. Ars. *99*, Aur. *109*.

weak and slow. Opium. *615/6*. Ver. vir. *858. 860*.

slow. Theridion. *815. 817*. Ver. vir. *859*. Cann. *183*, Cocc. *291*.

slow, with vertigo. Theridion. *817*.

rapid. Ail. *26, 28*. Ant. tart. *68*. Bapt. *114*. Bell. *121/2*. Camph. *176*. Glon. *388. 391*. Dros. *359*. Acon. *10*. Ars. *99*. Collin. *312*. Pyrogen *692. 695*.

almost pulseless. Ammon carb. *46*, Camph. *176*. Colch. *308*. Collin. *310*.

slow at rest, fast after

exertion. Arn. *90*.

weak, intermitting. Arn. *91*. Camph. *176*.

small, weak. Camph. *176*.

full, soft, flowing. Ferr. phos. *379. 380*.

< every movement. Ant. tart. *68*.

accelerated without fever. Camph. *176*.

< towards evening with orgasm of blood. Caust. *228*.

bounding. Acon. (Ferr. phos. *380*).

flowing. Gels. (Ferr. phos. *380*).

AS IF:

heart were enlarged. Sul. *780*.

heart were on right side. Borax. *137*.

heart would stop. Nux. mosch. *598*. Sepia *743*. Lob. Dig. Gels. *384*.

WITH:

difficulty in breathing on motion. Ammon. carb. *44*.

blueness of body. Carbo v. *213*, Lach. *492*.

icy coldness of whole surface. Carbo v. *213*.

cold sensation about . . . Nat. mur. *574*. Kali br. *460*.

dyspnoea. Colch. *305*.

pain down left arm and through to left shoulder blade. Crot. *337*. Theridion. *817*.

numbness of left arm and shoulder. Rhus. *710*.

cough. Ammon. carb . . . *44*.

squeezed feeling. Iod. (Gels *384*). Iod. *434*.

PALPITATIONS:

with great anxiety. Puls. *685*. Sul. *780*.

fluttering. Nat. mur. *574*. Sul. *780*.

acute. Acon. *7*. Ammon. carb. *45*, Ars. *99*. Cean. *233*. Ant. tart. *66*. Arg. nit. *80*, Ferr. *372*. Iod. *433*. Puls. Kali sul. *475*. Lil. tig. *509*, Ver. alb. *854*.

violent, audible. Ammon. carb. *45*. Bell. *116*. Con. *329*. Plat. *661*. Phos. *646*. Glon. *339/ 340*.

nervous. Asaf. *102*.

from over-exertion. Asaf. *102*.

from suppression of discharges. Asaf. *102*, Arn. Rhus. *710*.

trembling. Cicuta. *263*.

after any manual labour. Iod. *435*.

loud endocardial bruits. Aur. *109*.

violent and rapid on falling asleep. Sul. *780*.

< going upstairs or climbing a hill. Sul. *780*.

visible. Sul. *780*.

without anxiety, any time of the day. Sul. *780*.

< during stool. Sul. *780*.

< at night turning in bed. Sul. *780.*

tumultous beating. Tarent. *801.*

HEART DEPRESSANT IN PHYSIOLOGICAL DOSES.
Ver. vir. *859.* (note dangerous effect of slowing pulse rate in inflammatory diseases when a quickened pulse is salutary and is the normal response of the body to disease).

DROPSY OF THE HEART.
Aur. *108.*

CYANOSIS.
Carbo v. *213.* Ammon. carb. *44.*

HYPERTROPHY. Iod. *433. 435/6* Rhus. *710.*

HYDROPERICARDIUM. Colch. *309.*

PERICARDITIS.
Kali carb. *470.*

RHEUMATISM OF THE HEART.
Cimic. *274.* Kali carb. *472.*

CARDIALGIA.
Arg. nit. *80,* Staph. *763.*

RHEUMATIC AFFECTIONS THAT HAVE GONE TO THE HEART.
Aur. *108/9* Colch. *305.*

LIVER AILMENTS ASSOCIATED WITH THE HEART.
Aur. *108.*

ENDOCARDITIS.
Kali carb. *470.*

ENDOCARDITIS WITH PERICARDITIS.
Carbo v. followed by complementary remedy Kali carb. *472.*

HEART DISEASE FOLLOWING GOUT.
Colch. *309.*

HEART FAILURE.
Ammon. carb. *46.*

FATTY DEGENERATION.
Arn. *90,* Caps. *203,* Kali carb. *473.*

VALVULAR DISEASE.
Spig. Iod. *435.*

VALVULAR DISEASE FOLLOWING RHEUMATISM.
Colch. *305.*

ANXIETY AROUND HEART.
Acon. *10.* Colch. *305.* Psor. *677.*

> **LYING DOWN.**
Psor. *677.*

DILATION.
Ammon. carb. *44,* Rhus. *710.*
< going upstairs. Ammon. carb. *44.*
< in hot room. Ammon. carb. *44.*

INFLAMMATION RESULTING IN EFFUSION INTO PERICARDIUM.
Colch. *308.*

< **SLIGHTEST EXCITEMENT.**
Collin. *312.*

WEAK HEART WITH ABSENCE OF SYMPTOMS.
Ammon carb. *44/5.*

STRAIN AFTER EXERCISE.
Arn. *90*.

DIFFICULT BREATHING AS
RESULT OF CARDIAC
ATTACH.
Ammon. carb. *45* (single
dose).

WEAKNESS AND LOSS OF
BREATH GOING UPSTAIRS.
Iod. *433, 434*.

ALTERNATE CONGESTION TO
HEART AND TO HEAD.
Glon. *390*.

ALTERNATELY CONSTRICTED
AND RELEASED.
Lil. tig. (Gels. *384*).

BUZZING IN REGION OF HEART.
Cycl. *351*.

THROBBING CAROTID
ARTERIES.
Tarent. *799*.

MITRAL VALVES —
INSUFFICIENCY.
Kali carb. *473*.

< DURING OR AFTER SLEEP.
Lach. *492*.

PAIN IN PRECORDIAL REGION.
Lach. *498*. Sul. *790*, Tub. *834*.
Tarent *803*.

PULSATIONS SHAKE THE BODY.
Nat. mur. *573*.

METASTASIS FROM PAINS IN
LIMBS AND TOES.
Nat. phos. *577*.

THROBBING OF VESSELS OF
NECK.
Bell. Spig. Pyrogen *690*.

VIOLENT HEART'S ACTION.
Tarent. *808*, Pyrogen. *690*.

HARD LOUD HEART'S BEATS.
Pyrogen. *690*.

SENSATION OF SOMETHING
ALIVE IN . . .
Cycl. *351*.

SENSATION OF HEART
CONSTRICTED AS BY AN IRON
BAND.
Cactus (Gels. *384*). Nux
mosch. *598*, Lil. tig. *509, 512*.
Lil. tig. Iod. *433. 435*.

HEARTBURN
Caps. *200*.

WITH STOMACH PAIN.
Ammon. carb. *42*, Ant. crud.
55. Nux. v. *608*.

WITH ACIDITY.
Nat. phos. *576*.

WITH BLOATING.
Nux. v. *601*.

HELMINTHIASIS
WORMS. See WORMS.

HEMICRANIA
HEADACHE LIMITED TO ONE
SIDE OF THE HEAD. See
HEAD and
HEADACHES.

HEPATITIS
INFLAMMATION OF THE LIVER.
See LIVER.

HERNIA

FROM INACTIVITY OF RECTUM.
Cham. *240*.

LEFT-SIDED INGUINAL.
Cocc. *291*.

INCLINATION TO HERNIAS.
Cocc. *293, 296*. Nux. v. *605*.
< rising from sitting. Cocc.
296.

**TENDENCY TO INGUINAL
HERNIAS.**
Nux. v. *605* Tereb. *812*.

**INCARCERATED OR
STRANGULATED HERNIAS.**
Plumbum. *666*.

HERPES

ZOSTER (SHINGLES).
Ars. *94*. Iris *449*. *Mez*. *555*.
Variolinum. Ran. b. *698. 700*.

WITH INFLAMMATION.
Bell. *116*.

ERUPTIONS:
round mouth. Nat. mur.
Rhus. Sepia *743* Nat. mur.
573. Rhus (Cham *243*). Nat.
mur., Sepia. Borax *132*.

round nipples. Caust. *228*.

on lips. Nat. mur. *570,* Rhus.
Sepia *743*.

on thighs and arms. Nat. mur.
572.

between fingers. Nitric ac.
592.

from temple, over ears to
cheeks. Psor. *677*.

in bends of joints. Psor. *677*.

anywhere. Thuja. *820*.

on perineum. Pet. *633*.

CIRCINATUS.
Calc. *160*.

NEURALGIA AFTER . . .
Mez. *555*. Thuja. *820*.

BURNING > HEAT.
Ars. (Ran. b. *698*).

HICCOUGHS

Cicuta. *262/3 269*, Hyos. *414*.
Mag. phos. *525*. Ign. *430*. See
THROAT.

AFTER A MEAL.
Cycl. *350*.

FREQUENT.
Merc. *542*. Ran. b. *701*. Staph.
763.

VERY VIOLENT.
Stram. *777*.

ALMOST CONSTANT.
Ver. vir. *861*.

WHEN SMOKING TOBACCO.
Puls. *684*.

IN PNEUMONIA.
Ver. vir. *858*.

**WITH SPASMS IN UPPER END OF
OESOPHAGUS.**
Ver. vir. *861*.

AFTER EATING AND DRINKING.
Ign. *430*.

HODGKIN'S DISEASE

LYMPHADENOMA.
Cistus *288*.

HOME SICKNESS

Caps. *200, 202, 204*.

HOUSEMAID'S KNEE
Ruta 717.

HUNGER
HUNGRY YET LOSES FLESH.
Nat. mur. Acet. ac. Iodum.
Sanic. Tub. Abrot 3.

RABID OR EXCESSIVE HUNGER.
Alum. 37. Ammon carb. 43.
Bry. 149. Calc. 161.

EASILY SATISFIED.
Ammon. carb. 43.

HYDRAEMIA
EXCESS OF WATER IN THE
BLOOD.
Nat. sul. 580.

HYDROCELE
COLLECTION OF FLUID IN SAC
ENCLOSING TESTICLES OR
SPERMATIC CORD. See
GENITALIA.

HYDROCEPHALUS
FLUID ON THE BRAIN.
Arn. 91. Calc. p. 156, 159/60
167.

HYDROMETRA
DROPSY OF UTERUS,
ACCUMULATION OF WATERY
MUCOUS FLUID IN CAVITY OF
THE WOMB.
Colch. 309.

HYDROPHOBIA
FEAR OF WATER.
rabies. Bell. 120, Cann. 188.

192. Canth. 196. Hyos. 412.
409. Stram. 768.

HYDROTHORAX
COLLECTION OF DROPSICAL
FLUID IN THE PLEURAL
CAVITIES. See CHEST.

HYGROMA PATELLAE
Arn. 90.

HYPERAEMIA
CONGESTION OF BLOOD OR AN
EXCESSIVE AMOUNT IN A
PART.
Calc. 159. Canth. 194. Ferr.
phos. 379. 381. Glon. 391.
Ptelea 680.

HYPERAESTHESIA
See SENSITIVITY

HYPERINOSIS
Arn. 90.

HYPOCHONDRIUM
Brom. 141. Calc. 161. Cean.
231, Chel. 250. See
ABDOMEN.

I

ICTHYOSIS
FISH SCALE SURFACE TO SKIN.
See SKIN.

ICTERUS
JAUNDICE.
Plumbum. 665.

110

INFLAMMATIONS
OF:

eyes. Abrot. *1*. Acon. *5. 9*.

windpipe (croup. laryngitis)
Acon. *7*.

throat. Acon. *7*.

bladder. Acon. *7*. Canth. *195*.

lung and pleura. Bry. Phos.
Bell. *116. 119*.

brain. Bell. *119*.

liver. Bell. *119*.

breasts. Bell. *125*.

gastro-intestines. Canth. *194*.

genito-urinary mucous
membranes. Canth. *194*.

cut, becoming green and
odourous. Brom. *139*.

WITH:

heat, dry skin. Acon. *11*.

violent thirst. Acon. *11*.

red or alternating red and
pale face. Acon. *11*.

INTENSE.
Bell. *125*. Merc. cor. Ars.
Canth. *193*.

OF JOINTS WITH EXCESSIVE
HYPERAESTHESIA.
Colch. *309*.

CEASE, FOLLOWED BY
CONVULSIONS, DELIRIUM.
Cup. *345*.

AT OUTSET.
Ferr. phos. *379*.

SUPPURATING WHEN PUS IS
ABOUT TO OR IIAS ALREADY
FORMED.
Hepar *402/3*.

CHRONIC.
Sil. *756*.

INTERTRIGO
CHAFING OF SKIN. E.G. UNDER
BREAST OR IN ARMPIT.
See SKIN.

INTUSSUSCEPTION
OBSTRUCTION IN BOWELS
Plumbum. *664*.

IRON
AS TISSUE SALT.
Ferr. phos (Ferr. *369*).

CONSTITUENT OF MUSCLE
CELLS.
Ferrum. phos (Ferrum. *369*).

OXYGEN ATTRACTANT.
Ferrum. *369*.

SLEEPING IN MAGNETIC FIELD.
Ferr. *374*.

ISCHURIA
SUPPRESSION OR RETENTION OF
URINE IN BLADDER.
Arn. *89*.

ISOPATHY
Psor *671*.

J

JAUNDICE
Chel. 247. Iod. *434*.

CAUSED BY FEAR.
Acon. *4*.

CAUSED BY RAGE OR ANGER.
Acon. *4.* Cham. *237,* Nat. sul. *585.*

YELLOWNESS.
Lach. Crot. *335.* Phos. *644.*

MALIGNANT.
Crot. *335. 337.*

SUDDEN ATTACKS.
Crot. *338.*

FROM DEFICIENCY OF BILE.
Iris. *452.*

WITH PAIN IN REGION OF LIVER.
Nitric ac. *591.*

WITH HYPERAEMIA OF LIVER.
Ptelea. *680.*

JOINTS

PAINS:
tearing pains in . . . Bell. *122.* Kali bich. *455.*

flying from place to place. Bell. *125.* Colch. *303. 305,* Kali bich. *455.*

pale swelling, burning pains. Ars. *97.*

rheumatic. Caust *223,* Colch. *305.* Dros. *359.* Mag. phos. *525.*

in . . . Caust. *223,* Colch. *338.*

in all joints. Ipec. *446.*

in wrist joint. Bry. *150.*

SWELLING OF . . .
Aur. *109,* Bell. *125,* Bry. *150,* Caust. *223.*

SHRIVELLING.
Caust. *223.*

STIFFNESS IN . . .
Caust. *223,* Ledum. *501. 507,* Cocc. *297.* Colch. *303. 309.*

CRACKING IN . . .
Cham. *241,* Cocc. *297.* Pet. *630. 632.*

INFLAMED.
Colch. *303. 305.*

INFLAMED, WITH EXCESSIVE HYPERAESTHESIA.
Colch. *309.*

INFLAMMATION OF PERIOSTEUM.
Aur. *109.*

HOT, RED AND BURNING.
Bell. *125.* Colch. *309.*

THICKENING AND INDURATION OF PERIOSTEUM.
Aur. *109.*

PUFFY, BUT LITTLE RED.
Ferr. phos. *380.*

SMALL JOINTS AFFECTED.
Colch. *309,* Ledum. *502*

FISSURES IN BENDS.
Caust. *224.*

IN RHEUMATIC FEVER.
Bell. *125.*

> COLD WATER.
Ledum. 501. 507.

> HEAT.
Ars. (Ledum. *501*).

< MOVING.
Ledum. *502.*

< LYING DOWN.
Ledum. *502.*

FEELS AS IF WATER TRICKLING
INTO . . .
Nat. mur. *574.*

SYNOVIAL CREPITATION.
Nat. phos. *577.*

FATTY DEGENERATION OF . . .
Picric ac. *655.*

WEAKNESS IN . . .
Psor *677* Sepia. *747.*

EASILY SPRAINED.
Psor *677.*

STIFFNESS AND SENSE OF
FATIGUE IN ALL JOINTS.
Staph. *765.*

ARTHRITIC NODES ON . . .
Staph. *765.*

K

KERATITIS

INFLAMMATION OF CORNEA IN
FRONT OF EYE. See EYES.

KIDNEYS

PAIN:
    violent Calc. p. *168,* Canth.
    198, Colch. *307,* Tereb. *811.*
    cutting. Canth. *198.*
    burning. Canth. *198,* Tereb.
    810. 814.
    sticking . . . Mez. *553.*
    sharp stinging pain in region
    of kidneys. Kali bich. *458.*
    alternating with pain in penis.
    Canth. *198.*
    alternating with cloudy and
    drunken feeling. Alum. *37.*

THROBBING AND THUMPING
OVER SUPRARENALS.
Med. *535.*

ACUTE DISEASE WITH DROPSY.
Acon. 7 (followed by 'chronic'
Sulphur).

SUPPURATING.
Calc. s. *172.*

CONGESTED.
Canth. *194.*

ACUTE NEPHRITIS.
Canth. *194,* Colch. *309,* Lyc.
515. Arn. *89. 90.*

RENAL IRRITATION.
Chel. *249.*

INCREASED URIC ACID.
Chel. *249.*

ACHING BEFORE AND AFTER
URINATION.
Lyc. *518.*

BUBBLING SENSATION IN . . .
Med. *531.*

CREEPING CHILL.
Med. *535.*

CONTRACTED.
Plumbum *667/8.*

BRIGHT'S DISEASE.
Plumbum. *668.*

INTERSTITIAL INFLAMMATION.
Plumbum. *669.*

PYELITIS.
Stram. *779.*

RENAL CONGESTION.
Tereb. 814.

KOUMISS
Calc. p. *169.*

L

LANDRY'S DISEASE
Cocc. *294*.

LARYNGISMUS STRIDULUS
SPASMODIC CROUP. See CROUP.

LARYNX
LARYNGITIS.
Acon. *5*. Allium *31*. Ant. tart. *68*, Dros. *352*.

CATARRHAL LARYNGITIS.
Aesc. *15*.

INFLAMED.
Bell. *122*. Allium. *31*.

SWOLLEN.
Bell. *122*, Iod. *434*, Lach. *498*.

ROUGHNESS IN . . .
Carbo v. *212*. Phos. *645*.

CONSTRICTED.
Cham. *241*, Iod. *434*. Ver. alb. *855*.

SENSATION OF RAWNESS AND SCRAPING.
Cham. *241*, Dros. *361*.

HOARSENESS > HAWKING.
Cham. *241*, Phos. *645*.

LARYNGEAL PHTHISIS.
Dros. *352*.

LARYNGITIS OF SINGERS.
Ferr. phos. *379*.

SPASM OF GLOTTIS.
Iod. *434*, Chlorine (Iod. *435*).

ROPY DISCHARGES IN LARYNGITIS.
Kali bich. *456*.

THICK MEMBRANE IN . . .
Kali bich. *456*.

DEGENERATION OF MUCOUS MEMBRANES IN . . .
Kreos. *478*.

COUGH IMPELS PATIENT TO GRASP LARYNX.
Allium *31*.

DRY AND STIFF.
Aesc. *15*. Bell. *122*. Con. *327*.

LOOSE RATTLING.
Brom. *139*. *141/2*.

SENSATION OF COLDNESS.
Brom. *141*.

SENSITIVE TO COLD AIR.
Hepar *407*.

WITH DEEP ROUGH VOICE.
Carbo. v. *212*.

MUSCLES REFUSE TO FUNCTION.
Caust. *228*.

MUCOUS IN . . .
Cina *283*, Hyos *414*.

CHRONIC ITCHING IN . . .
Cistus *287*.

LOUD WHEEZING.
Cistus *287*.

VIOLENT TICKLING IN . . .
Cocc. *297*, Iod. *434*.

TICKLING IN . . .
leading to cough. Dros. *355*, *361*, Psor. *677*

FLUIDS GO DOWN . . .
Hyos. *412*.

DISTURBANCE.
Ign. *428.*

DESIRE TO COUGH, BUT >
SUPPRESSING COUGH.
Ign. *431.*

VIOLENT SPASMS.
Ant. crud. *55,* Ign. *428.* Vib. *864.*

LASSITUDE OF WHOLE BODY
Alum. *38/9.*

LAUGHTER UNCONTROLLABLE
Cann. *182. 184.*

LAW OF SIMILARS
Calc. p. *169,* Dros. *361.*

LEGS
PAIN:
in tibia < at night. Asaf. *102. 104.* Dros. Asaf. *104.*

in long bones. Dros. Asaf. *104.* Dros. *352.*

in calf, ankle joints. < motion. Bry. *144.*

in ankle joint. Dros. *361,* Ledum. *505.*

tensive pain in knees. Caps. *202,* Caust. *229* Iod. *434.* Ledum. *505.*

drawing, tearing pain in thighs, legs, knees & feet. Caust *229.* Chel. *251.*

in right knee < moving. Chel. *251.*

in achilles tendon when walking. Cocc. *298.*

cramp-like in thighs. Cycl. *351.*

bruised, in knee joint. Ars. *94.*

bruised, in legs. Nux. mosch. *599.*

stitching pain in calf > walking. Dros. *361.*

in all bones. Dros. *361.*

inflamed knees. Nat. phos. *575*

aching pain in . . . Rhus. *713.*

< in open air. Caust. *229.*

> warmth of bed. Caust *229.*

piercing pains in swollen knees. Sal. ac. *725.*

gonagra. Caust. *229.*

ANKLES:
sprained. Ledum. *506,* Pet. *629.* Rhus *711.* Ruta *717.*

itching with eczema. Nat. phos. *578.*

ankle joints stiff. Sul. *790.*

pricking, itching. Staph. *764.*

CALVES:
rigidity in . . . Arg. nit. *80.*

spasms and cramps in . . . Cup *346*

tearing in muscles of . . . Staph. *764.*

cramp in . . . Sul. *790.*

KNEES:
constant cold knees in bed. Phos. *647.*

115

stiff and cracking. Sul. *790*.

pain under knees. Ver. alb. *855*.

hot knees, with cold nose. Ign. *430*.

stiffness in . . . < motion. Bry. *144. 150*.

cold. Carbo v *207, 211, 213*. Nat. mur. *569*.

cracking in . . . Caust. *229*, Cocc. *297*.

trembling of . . . Ledum. *505*.

weakness in . . . Cocc. *292, 297.*, Ledum. *505*.

knees strike together. Colch. *309*.

grasping sensation in . . . Nux. mosch. *598*.

swelling of . . . Calc. *162*, Hepar *405*, Ledum. *504/5*

> cold. Ledum. *504, 507*.

AS IF BONE FROM KNEE TO ANKLE HAD BEEN SMASHED.
Nux. mosch. *598*.

AS IF BONES IN LEG WERE DECAYING.
Sepia. *744*.

COLD BELOW KNEES, IN WARM ROOM.
Sil. *755*.

IRRITABLE STUMP AFTER OPERATION.
Symphitum. *797*.

STAGGERING GAIT AS IF DRUNK.
Tereb. *813*.

PERIOSTITIS.
Agar. Lach. Rhus. Dros. Asaf. *104*. Phos. *646*.

AS IF BRUISED ALL OVER.
Bell. *122*.

WEAK AND PROSTRATED.
Brom. *140*.

WEAKNESS IN THIGHS.
Bry. *150*. Cina *283*, Cocc. *292*, Mur. ac. *566*.

WEAKNESS IN LEGS.
Bry. *150*. Calc. *162*. Cocc. *292*. Con. *331*. Picric ac. *657*. Rhus. *712*.

< from study. Picric ac. *657*.

< from walking. Rhus. *713*.

WEAKNESS IN 'LOWER EXTREMITIES'.
Rhus. *715*.

LEGS WEAK GOING UP OR DOWN STAIRS.
Ruta. *721*.

TREMBLING.
Cimic. *273*. Mag. phos. *525*.

UNABLE TO WALK EXCEPT BY SPRINGS INVOLVING BOTH LEGS.
Ver. vir. *862*.

RESTLESSNESS AND WEARINESS OF . . .
Ruta. *721*. Colch. *304*.

HEAVINESS BY DAY.
Puls. *685*. Rhus. *713/4*. Ver. alb. *855*.

TENSION IN KNEES AND FEET.
Rhus. *714*

STITCHES IN KNEE JOINT
< MOVEMENT.
Staph. *764.*

STITCHES IN TIBIA.
Staph. *764.*

EXHAUSTION IN . . . WHEN
WALKING.
Phos. ac. *638.*

TWITCHES.
Anac. *49*, Mez. *554.*

PAGET'S DISEASE.
Dros. Asaf. *104.*

CRAMP.
Colch. *304*, Mag. phos. *525.*

LAMENESS AFTER SUPPRESSED
SWEAT.
Colch. *308.*

ASCENDING PARALYSIS.
Con. *331.*

LIMBS FEEL BRUISED.
Dros. *361.*

FEEL PARALYZED.
Dros. *361.*

'GONE TO SLEEP' FEELING.
Ign. *431.* Ledum. *506.*

PITTING ON PRESSURE.
Ledum. *506.*

COLD.
Nat. mur. *569.*

SYPHILITIC NODES ON SHIN
BONES.
Nitric ac. *592.*

TOTTERING GAIT.
Ail. *27*, Alum. *38.*

SCIATICA.
Arn. *90.* Cimic. *271.* Abrot. 1.
Mag. phos. *525.* Rhus. *711.*

cured by mechanical
treatment. Aesc. *13.*

through lump on femur. Ferr.
Aesc. *13.*

left sided. Clinicum. (*Med.
535*).

< on lying down at night.
Ruta. *720.*

< motion. Bry. *144.*

LEUCOPHLEGMATIC
Calc. *154. 159.*

LEUCOPLAKIA
HARD, SMOOTH, WHITISH
PATCHES ON TONGUE – See
TONGUE.

LEUCORRHEA
YELLOW.
Kreos. *479.* Sepia *742.* Vib.
865. Kali bich. *460.* Cham.
240. Iod. *435.*

DARK YELLOW, THICK, STICKY.
Aesc. *14*, Calc. *162.* Cean. *235.*

WHITE OR STARCHY.
Borax. *135.* Graph. *399.*
Kreos. *479.*

LIKE WHITE OF EGG.
Borax. *135.*

LIKE MILK.
Calc. *161/2*

GREENISH.
Merc. *543.* Thuja. Nat. sul.
581.

PROFUSE.
Alum. *39.* Calc. *161.*

ACRID.
Ammon. carb. *45*. Ars. *94*.
Borax *136*. Graph. *399*.

EXCORIATING.
Caul. *219*, Graph. *399*. Iod.
435. Kreos *482*. Mez. *553*

CHRONIC.
Iod. *432*.

ROPY DISCHARGES.
Kali bich. *456. 460*.

PUTRID.
Kreos. *472. 482*. Psor *673, 677*.

SOUR SMELLING.
Nat. phos. *576*.

CARRION-LIKE ODOUR.
Psor. *678*.

STRONG, OFFENSIVE ODOUR.
San. *732*. Hepar *402*, Kreos
482, Tereb. *810*.

ODOUR OF FISH BRINE.
San. *735*.

WITH:
itching and burning. Calc.
161.
great debility. Calc. *162*.
stinging in os and in vagina.
Calc. *162*.
burning in cervical canal.
Calc. *162*.
chlorosis. Calc. *162*.
pruritus. Calc. *162*.
bearing down pains. Caul.
216.
violent pains in sacrum. Psor.
677.
backache. Mur. ac. *564*.

BEFORE AND AFTER MENSES.
Calc. *161*.

DURING MICTURITION.
Calc. *161/2*.

< AFTER EXERCISE.
Calc. *162*.

IN SCROFULOUS WOMEN.
Calc. *162*.

< BY DAY.
Calc. *162*.

BLOODY.
Tereb. *810*.

< IN AFTERNOON.
Iod. *432*.

LIEUTERY
China. *258*.

LIMBS
PAINS:
violent in extremities.
Plumbum. *669*.
in both hip joints. Rhus. *713*.
in limbs on which lain. Rhus.
713.
as from blow or fall. Ruta. *721*.
as if bruised. Ruta *721*
side of body lain on feels
painful. Sil. *754*. Ruta
(Symphitum *794*).
in thighs on walking. Staph.
764.
in all bones. Staph. *764*.
in small spots when touched.
Ign. *431*
< at night. Puls. Kali sul. *475*.
< warmth. Puls. Kali sul. *475*.

118

> cold open air. Puls. Kali
sul. *475.*

start in lower limbs and travel
upwards. *Ledum. 501.*

start in higher limbs and
travel down. Kalmia (Ledum.
501).

in shoulder joints. Ledum.
505.

< movement. Ledum. *505.*

move from limb to heart.
Benzoic. ac. Nat. phos. *578.*

drawing pains all over. Nitric
ac. *592.*

cramp-like, < pressure. Plat.
661.

in right hip. Nat. sul. *585.*

in right thigh, only when
walking. Coloc. *319.*

in loins and thighs. Dulc. *366.*

in left hip joint. Ant. crud. *54.*

in loins and thighs. Dulc. *366.*

extending from fingers or toes
towards the body. Hyp. *418.*

wandering. Tub. *835.*

< standing. Tub. *835.*

> continued motion. Tub.
835.

with lameness and numbness.
Agar. *25.*

burning, lancinating in foot.
Ant. crud. *56.*

tensive, shooting pain in loin.
Coloc. *319.*

in hip joint. Dros. *361.*

drawing pains. Hepar. *405.*

LIMBS ON WHICH HE LIES FEEL
SORE.
Arn. Nux mosch. *598.*

NEURALGIA IN . . .
Chel. *251.* Coloc. *314.*
Plumbum. *669.*

DISTORTION.
Cicuta. *263.*

PARALYSIS.
Caust. *223, 229.* Con. *329.*

CONTRACTION OF . . .
Abrot. *2.*

> HANGING DOWN.
Con. *323. 329.*

LOSS OF POWER.
Con. *329.*

YELLOW.
Crot. *336.*

LOSS OF CONTROL.
Gels. *386.*

PUNCTURED WOUNDS IN . . .
Ledum. (Hyp. *418*).

BRUISING OR LACERATING OF
NERVE ENDS.
Hyp. *418.*

INJURED 'SOFT' PARTS.
Arn. (Hyp. *419*).

INJURED NERVES.
Hyp. *419.*

LACERATED WOUNDS.
Hyp. *419.*

TO HEAL LIP OF WOUNDS.
Hyp. *419.*

NUMBNESS IN ARMS AT NIGHT.
Arg. nit. *83.*

JERKING ON GOING TO SLEEP.
Ifn. *431.*

FEELING AS IF LIMBS
ENLARGED.
Ant. crud. *55.*

BLUISH SPOTS ON THIGHS AND
TIBIA.
Ant. crud. *56.*

BLACK FOOT.
Ant. crud. *56.*

BRUISED FEELING IN ANY LIMB.
Arnica 84. Ledum. *507,* Merc.
543. Phos. ac. *638.*

SPRAINED FEELING IN ANY
LIMBS.
Arn. *84.*

RESTLESS, HAS TO CHANGE
POSITION OF HIS FEET.
Ars. *100.*

UNDULATING TWITCHING OF
MUSCLES.
Asaf. *105.* Rhus. *715.*

CRAMP.
Calc. *155.*

DEFORMED.
Calc. *156.*

COLD.
Camph. *176,* Carbo v. *211,*
Ledum. *506.*

ICY COLDNESS.
Calc. *155.*

SEEM ENLARGED.
Cann. *179.*

> REST.
Cann. *179.*

PARALYSIS OF LOWER
EXTREMITIES.
Cann. *183.* Con. *329.* Cocc.
297.

'THRILLING' IN ARMS, HANDS,
LOWER LEGS.
Cann. *183.*

CLUMSY.
Carbo v. *207.*

AFTER MANIPULATION OF
PELVIS.
Ruta *719.*

BODY ODOUR VERY OFFENSIVE.
Psor. *675.*

PUFFY, PURPLE AND COLD.
Ledum. *501.*

PUFFY, PURPLE AND HOT.
Lach. (Ledum. *501*).

SHAKING.
Mag. phos. *525.*

AS IF FLOATING IN AIR.
Nux. mosch. *598.*

HEAVINESS IN LOWER LIMBS.
Alum. *36.* Gels. *382.* Arg. nit.
80. Bry. *150.* Chel. *251.*

STAGGERS.
Alum. *36.* Arg. nit. *80.*

WEARINESS OF ALL LIMBS.
Con. *329.* Gels. *386.* Merc. *543.*

WEARINESS OF LEGS WHEN
SITTING.
Alum. *36.* Bry. *150.*

GENERAL DEBILITY WITH
TREMBLING.
Arg. nit. *80.* Gels. *384.*

EXCESSIVE WEAKNESS AND
EXHAUSTION OF LIMBS.
Ars. *99.*

TREMULOUS WEAKNESS.
Arg. nit. *81.* Brom. *140.* Con.
329. Cimic. *272.* Cann. *179.*

Chel. *251*, Gels. *386*. Opium.
613. *616*. Picric ac. *657*.
Viscum *868*.

EASILY FATIGUED.
Gels. *386*.

FORMICATION OF LOWER LIMBS.
Aeth. *20*, Alum. *39*.

WEAKNESS.
Caust. *229*. Con. *329*. Phos.
646. Sil. *753*.

TREMBLING IN ARMS AND
LOWER EXTREMITIES.
Rhus. *713*. Stram. *775*.

WEARY — LEADING TO
PARALYSIS.
Picric ac. *657*.

BRUISED FEELING ALL OVER
AFTER COITION.
Sil. *754*.

LACKING POWER OR STABILITY
IN THIGHS.
Ruta *721*.

BUTTOCKS — PRICKLING
ITCHING MUSCLES.
Staph. *764*.

RESTLESS LIMBS.
Pyrogen. Rhus. *714*. Stram.
775.

STIFF ON FIRST MOVING LIMB
AFTER REST.
Rhus. *713/4*.

STIFF AND PARALYSED.
Rhus. *712*.

HIP JOINTS PARALYSED.
Ver. alb. *855*.

CANNOT BEAR LIMBS TO TOUCH
EACH OTHER AT NIGHT.
Psor. *672*.

ACHING ALL OVER.
Pyrogen *692*

FIBROUS TISSUES AFFECTED.
Rhod. *706*. Rhus. *711*. *715*.

SEROUS TISSUES AFFECTED.
Bry. (Rhod. *706*).

FRACTURES.
Symphitum *794*.

FRACTURES THAT FAIL TO
UNITE.
Symphitum. *794*.

LIPOMATA ON THIGHS.
Baryta carb. Pet. *628*.

HIP DISEASE.
Phos ac. *639*.

BRUISE EASILY.
Phos. *643*.

EXTREMITIES COLD.
Picric ac. *657*.

NUMBNESS HERE AND THERE.
Plat. *661*.

PARALYSIS OF EXTENSORS,
FOREARM OR UPPER LIMB
WITH EXCESSIVE
HYPERAESTHESIA OR
PARTIAL ANAESTHESIA.
Plumbum. *667*.

LIME
Calc. *157*.

LIPOMATA
FATTY TUMOURS.
Pet. *628*. See LIMBS.

LIPS

BLUISH OR PURPLISH FROM LACK OF OXYGEN.
Ant. tart. Arn. Ammon carb. *44*

BRIGHT.
red. Sul. *787.*

RED AND BLEEDING.
Kreos *484.*

BLEEDING.
Lach. *499.*

BURNING.
Tub. Sul. *782/3.*

LIVID.
Camph. *176.*

ROUGH.
Sul. *788.*

TINGLING.
Picric ac. *657.*

SWELLING.
Hepar *405,* Lach. *497.* Asaf. *102.* Psor. *676.* Nat. mur. *572*

RAW, DRY, SCABBY.
Ammon. carb. *45.* Sul. *788.*

DRY.
Ant. crud. *53.* Bry. *145.* Cann. *182.* Lach. *499.* Ver. vir. *861.* Sul. *788.*

PARCHED AND CRACKED.
Bapt. *114.* Lach. *499.*

CHAPPED.
Calc. *160.* Caps. *200.*

CRACKED.
Calc. *160,* Ign. *430.* Sul. *788.*

NUMB.
Nat. mur. *574.*

FISSURES.
Caust. *224.*

CRACK IN CENTRE OF LOWER LIP.
Nat. mur. Sep. Graph. Cham *239.* Dros. Sepia. *740.*

CRACK IN MIDDLE OF LOWER LIP.
Nat. mur. *569, 572.*

SCABS ON UPPER LIP.
Arum. tryph. San. *733.*

TINGLING AS OF CRAWLING OF ANTS.
Picric ac. *657.*

'GLUED TOGETHER'.
Cann. *182.*

SORDES ON LIPS.
Bapt. *115.*

EPITHELIOMA.
Cicuta *265.*

SALIVA EXCORIATING.
Ammon. carb. *45.*

PAIN IN RIGHT LOWER LIP.
Phos. ac. *637.*

LITHOTOMY

OPERATION FOR STONES IN BLADDER.
Staph. *763.*

LIVER

PAINS IN:
Allium *32,* Chel. *250.* Con. *328.* Crot. *337,* Lyc. *518.* Nat. sul. *584.* Ptelea *679.*

in left hypogastrium. Allium *32.* Lyc. *518.* Ptelea *679.*

with urging to urinate. Allium *32.*

with scalding urine. Allium *32.*

stitching. movement. Bry. *144,* Chel. *250.*

with fixed pain under lower angle of right shoulder blade *Chel. 246. 249.*

shooting towards back. Chel. *250.*

< after anger. Cocc. *291. 298.*

< lying on right side. Mag. mur. (Ptelea *680*).

< motion. Iris. *452.*

< lying on left side. Nat. sul. *585,* Ptelea *679.* Bry. Ptelea *680.*

TENDERNESS OVER.
Ail. *28,* Ferr. *372,* Nat. sul. *584/5* Ptelea *679* Ruta *720.*

CONGESTION OF . . .
Aloe, Collin. Nux. v. Sul., Pod., Aesc. *14.* Merc. *535.* Ptelea *679.*

HEPATITIS.
Chel. *250/1.* Phos. *644.* Ptelea. *679.*

FATTY LIVER.
Chel. *251.*

ENLARGEMENT OF . . .
Chel. *251,* Cocc. *291.* Con. *322.* Mag. mur. (Ptelea *680*). Ferr. *372.* Nat. sul. *585,* Ptelea *679.*

HARDNESS IN REGION OF . . .
Graph. *399.*

SORE TO TOUCH.
Iod. *434.*

SCLEROSIS OF . . .
Nat. phos. *576.*

HEPATIC FORM OF DIABETES.
Nat. phos. *576.*

FATTY DEGENERATION OF . . .
Picric ac. *655.*

AFTER OEDEMA OF FEET AND LEGS SET IN.
Ptelea. *680.*

LOCHIA
DISCHARGE AFTER CHILDBIRTH. See
PREGNANCY.

LOCKJAW
Hyp. *418.*

LOCOMOTOR ATAXIA
See SPINE and PARALYSIS

LOQUACITY
Cann. *180. 182. 188.* Cocc. *290.* Crot. *338.* Lach. *495.* Hyos. Lach. *496. 498.*

LUMBAGO
Cimic. *274.*

PAIN ATTEMPTING TO RISE.
Rhus. *710.*

> WARMTH.
Rhus. *710*

< COLD.
Rhus. *710.*

LUMBRICI
See WORMS.

LUNGS
OPPRESSED BREATHING.
Ars. 97.

FEELING AS IF LUNGS COULD
NOT BE FULLY EXPANDED.
Asaf. *102*.

FEEL TOO TIGHT.
Nat. mur. *574*.

GREAT EXPLOSIVE POWER.
Ipec. Ant. tart. *64*.

LACK OF EXPLOSIVE POWER.
Ant. tart. *64*.

ACCUMULATION OF MUCOUS
WITH COARSE RATTLING.
Ant. tart. 63.

MUST SIT UP TO BREATH.
Ant. tart. *62*, Ars. *97*.

WHEEZY AND FROTHY
EXPECTORATION.
Ars. *97*.

SUPPURATING.
Calc. s. *172*.

BURNING.
Canth. *195*, Phos. *644*.

INFLAMMATIONS.
Canth. *195*, Ferr. *372*. Nitric
ac. *589*.

HEPATIZATION.
Chel. *251*.

HAEMOPTYSIS.
Chel. *251*. Ipec. *446* Arn. *90*.
Ars. *94*. Kreos *483*. Ledum.
502. *507*. Nitric ac. *592*.

OEDEMA.
Ammon. carb. *44*, Ant. tart.
66. *68*.

SORE AND TENDER.
Ail. *28*.

ORTHOPNOEA.
Ant. tart. *62*. Carb. v. *213*.

ENGORGEMENT OF RIGHT
LUNG.
Chel. *248*.

AFFECTIONS OF RIGHT LUNG.
Elaps. (Crot. *337*).

AFFECTIONS OF BASE OF LEFT
LUNG.
Nat. sul. *580*.

AFFECTIONS OF UPPER THIRD
OF RIGHT LUNG.
Ars. (Sepia *742*).

AFFECTIONS OF CENTRAL
THIRD OF RIGHT LUNG.
Sepia *742*.

PAIN IN APEX TO BASE OF
LUNG.
Cimic. *273*.

HAEMORRHAGES AFTER
MECHANICAL INJURIES.
Ipec. *446*.

WITH YELLOW
EXPECTORATION.
Puls. Kali. sul. *475*.

GANGRENE OF . . .
Kreos. *478/9*.

GANGRENE, FOLLOWING LOBAR
PNEUMONIA.
Phos. *645*.

MUCOUS RALES IN BOTH LUNGS.
Phos. *646*.

BLOODY EXPECTORATION
FROM . . .
Phos. *646*.

TUBERCLES DEVELOP.
Phos. *646*.

CHRONIC BLENORRHEA OF
LUNGS.
Psor. *677.*

AS IF KNIFE IN TOP OF LEFT
LUNG.
Sepia *744.* Sul. *784.*

SUPPURATION. < LOOKING
INTO THE LIGHT.
Stram. *772.*

LEFT LUNG IRRITATED.
Bacillinum. (Tub. *834*) Tub.
837.

LEFT LUNG PAINFUL.
Tub. *835.*

IN PERSON WITH T.B. HISTORY.
Tub. *835.*

SENSITIVE TO COLD AIR.
Aesc. *15.*

LUPUS
Cistus. *288.*

LYMPHATIC CONSTITUTION
DISPOSITION TO LYMPH
ACCUMULATION.
Ammon. carb. *42. 43.*

SWELLING OF CERVICAL
LYMPHATICS.
Ammon. carb. *45.*

LYMPHATIC ENLARGEMENTS.
Calc. *156.* Iod. *436.*

M

MACULAE
SPOTS IN EYES. See EYES.

MALARIA
Arn. *90,* Pyrogen. *697.* Nat.
mur. *569.*

FEVER, CHILL. SWEAT ALL
ERRATIC.
Sepia. *749.*

FEVER, CHILL, SWEAT IN
ORDERLY CASES.
China. Nat. mur (Sepia *749*).

MAMMARY GLANDS
SWELLING.
Aeth. *20,* Calc. *162.* Con. *327.*
Phyt. 650.

SORE.
Calc. p. *168.* Con. *324.* Med.
531. Phyt. *650.*

HARD, BUT NOT RED.
Calc. *162.* Con. *324. 327.*

HARD AND TENDER.
Cham. *241,* Phyt. *651.*

INFLAMED.
Phyt. 650. Cistus *288.* Con. *329.*

SHRIVELLING.
Con. *327.*

INDURATED FOLLOWING
BREAST ABSCESS.
Con. *329.*

INDURATED FOLLOWING
BLOWS.
Bellis (Symphitum. *793*).

LUMPS IN BREAST.
Con. *329,* Kreos. *480,* Iod. *434.*
Lac. can. *488,* Thuja *824*

HYPERTROPHY OF BREAST.
Con. *329,* Med. *531.*

ATROPHY.
Con. *329*, Kreos. *480*. Iod. *434*.
436.

TUMOUR.
Iod. *434*, Merc. iod. flavus.
Merc. *540*.

HARD CIRRHUS-LIKE TUMOURS.
Con. *328*.

CANCER OF . . .
Graph. *400*. Kreos *482*.

MASTITIS.
Lac. can. *489*. Arn. *91*.

NIPPLES — CRACKED AND
EXCORIATED.
Phyt. *654*.
sore. Caust. *228*.

GLANDS FEEL TOO LARGE.
Calc. p. *168*. Iod. *434*.

INFRA-MAMMARY PAIN.
Cimic. *272*. *274*.

SHIVERING OVER MAMMAE.
Cocc. *298*.

PAINFUL DURING MENSES.
Con. *324*.

STITCHES AS OF NEEDLES.
Con. *328*.

NEED SUPPORT GOING UP OR
DOWN STAIRS.
Lac. can. *488/9*.

< LEAST JAR.
Bell. Lac. can. *488*.

COLD TO TOUCH.
Med. *531*.

MILK IN BREASTS OF NON
PREGNANT WOMEN.
Merc. *539*.

WITH STRINGY MILK.
Phyt. *650*.

PAIN STARTS FROM NIPPLE AND
RADIATES.
Phyt. *651*. *654*.

WITH ABSCESSES.
Phyt. *651*, *654*.

WITH ULCERS.
Phyt. *651*.

WITH HARD PAINFUL
NODOSITIES.
Phyt. *654*.

MARASMUS

PROGRESSIVE WASTING.
Abrot. *2*.

< LOWER EXTREMITIES.
Abrot. *2*.

< FROM MALNUTRITION.
Abrot. *2*.

FROM BELOW UPWARDS.
Abrot. *2*.

FROM ABOVE DOWNWARDS.
San. Nat. mur, Lyc. (Abrot.
3).

< IN NECK.
Nat. mur. *569*.

WITH ENLARGED ABDOMEN OF
CHILDREN DUE TO
DEFECTIVE ASSIMILATION.
Bar. carb. Sil. Nat. mur. SUl.
Calc. Iod. Abrot. *3*.

WITH HEAD SWEATS.
Calc. *156*.

MASTOID

SUPPURATION OF MASTOID
ANTRUM. See EARS.

MASTURBATION.
Bellis. *130.*

MEASLES
Puls. 687.

VERY DRY BARKING COUGH.
Acon. *11.*

LIVID. Ail. *27.*

RASH FAILS TO COME OUT.
Ail. *27.*

SUDDENLY RECEDING.
Ail. *27.*

CONGESTION OF CHEST
FOLLOWING . . .
Camph. *176.*

HAEMORRHAGIC.
Ferr. phos. *379.*

EYES ALMOST CLOSED,
SWOLLEN.
Gels. *383.*

WATERY YELLOWISH-GREEN
SECRETIONS.
Puls. Kali bich. *457.*

WITH CORYZA AND PROFUSE
LACHRYMATION.
Puls. Kali bich. *457.*

WITH PUSTULES ON CORNEA.
Kali bich. *457.*

NEVER WELL SINCE . . .
Morbillinum. 561.

MECHANICAL LESIONS
Aesc. *19.*

MEIBOMIAM GLAND
See EYES.

MEMORY
LACKING.
Acon. *9.*

WEAK.
Merc. *541, 545.* Staph. *761*
Acon. *9.* Arn. *88.* Caust. *226*
Colch. *307.* Med. *534.* Con.
321.

LOSS OF . . .
Ail. *27, Anac. 47* Kali br. *466*
Lyc. *515. 520.* Nat. sul. *582.*
Nux mosch. *596.* Phos. ac. *639.*
Plumbum. *668.* Rhod. *705.*

DISBURBANCE IN . . .
Arg. nit. *78.*

FORGETFULNESS.
Cann. *182* Con. *327.*

TEMPORARY LOSS OF . . .
Cicuta *265,* Con. *327.* Nat.
mur, Nux. mosch. (Cicuta
265).

ABSOLUTELY DESTROYED.
Kali br. *467.*

MENSES
SUPPRESSED.
Abrot. *2.* Cimic. *272.* Cycl.
350. Glon. *389.* Ver. vir. *861.*

DELAYED.
Cimic. *272.* Graph. *399.* Nux.
mosch. *597.*

SUPPRESSED MENSES RETURN.
Collin. *312.*

SUPPRESSED LEADING TO
GOITRE.
Ferr. *370.*

IRREGULAR.
Cimic *272,* Cocc. *291.* Nux.
mosch. *597.*

PALE AND SCANTY.
Alum. *39,* Cycl. *350,* Vib. *865.*

TOO SOON.
Bell. *122.* Calc. *161.* Caust.
225. Cocc. *297.* Kreos *483.*
Cycl. *350,* Ferr. *370.* Kali carb.
471. Phos. *645.* Tub. *837.* Calc.
155, Nux. v. *607.* Plat. *661.*

VERY PROFUSE.
Bell. *122.* Calc. *161.* Ferr. *370.*
Kreos *483.* Tub. *837.* Merc.
543, Nux. mosch. *597.* Plat.
660/1.

LAST TOO LONG.
Calc. *161* Ferr. *370.*

CEASE ON LYING DOWN.
Caust. *225.*

ONLY DURING THE DAY.
Caust. *225.*

ITCHING OF PUDENDA BEFORE.
Graph. *399.*

FLOW ON SITTING DOWN.
Kreos *483.*

PROFUSE AS RESULT OF LEAST
EXCITEMENT.
Calc. *161.*

EXCESSIVE LOSS OF BLOOD.
Ars. *94.*

TOO FEEBLE.
Caust. *225.*

WITH:
chorea. Cimic. *272.*
hysteria. Cimic *272.*
mental disease. Cimic. *272.*
distension of abdomen. Cocc.
297.

contracting pains in
adbomen. Cocc. *297.*

contraction of rectum. Cocc.
297.

ringing in ears, Ferr. *370.*

headaches and vertigo. Cycl.
350. Kreos. *479.*

pain in the back. Nux. mosch.
597.

unconquerable drowsiness.
Nux. mosch. *597.*

cramp in abdomen. Nux. v.
607.

cramp-like colic pains. Vib.
864.

nausea in morning. Nux. v.
607. Vib. *864.*

CHILLINESS AND ATTACKS OF
FAINTING.
Nux. v. *607.*

COLD AS DEATH, LIPS AND
EXTREMITIES BLUE DURING.
Ver. alb. *856.*

PAINFUL PRESSING DOWN.
Plat. *661.*

ODOUR — CARRION-LIKE.
Psor *678.*

THICK AND BLACK.
Plat. *660.*

CONDITIONS < MENSES.
Cimic. *277.*

WITH DELIRIUM AT ONSET.
Cocc. *291.*

VICARIOUS MENSTRUATION BY
NOSEBLEED.
Bry. *147.*

MENTALS

ABSENT-MINDED.
Cann. *182*, Hepar *206*, Lac.
can. *488*. Phos. ac. *636*. Med.
534.

ALWAYS IN A HURRY.
Med. *534*, Lil. tig. *509* Arg. nit
(Lil. tig. *510*).

ANTHROPHOBIC.
Cicuta *261*, *264*. Dros. Cycl.
351.

ANXIOUS.
Caust. *222*, Cicuta. *261*. Iod.
434.

**ADVERSE TO SOCIETY, YET
DREADS TO BE ALONE.**
Con. *321*, Lyc. *514*.

CHANGEABLE.
San. *732*. Tarent. *801*.

CONFUSED.
Alum. *39*. Glon. *389*, Lach.
499. Alum. *39*, *40*. Lyc. *516*.
Lac. can. *490*. Mez. *552*, Anac.
Bapt. *113*. Bell. *124*. Bry. *148*.
Calc. *155*. *158*. Caps. *200*.

CONSCIENCE STRICKEN.
Staph. Cycl. *351*.

CONTEMPT FOR OTHERS.
Plat. *658*.

CROSS, UGLY, IRRITABLE.
Cham. Nux. v. Cina. Staph.
766.

CRUEL, NO HUMANITY.
Abrot. *1*.

**DISCONTENTED WITH
EVERYTHING.**
Pall. *626*.

DISINCLINED TO SPEAK.
taciturn. Glon. *388*, Hyos. *413*.
Phos. ac. *636/7*. Phos. *645*,
Picric ac. *656*. Sepia *745*.
Tarent *800* Lach. *496 ! !* Lyc.
521.

DISCINCLINED TO WORK.
Nat mur. *572*. Phos. *641*, Picric
ac. *656*. Sang. *729*. Sul. *786*.

DULL AND UNINSPIRING.
Con. *321*.

EGOTISTIC.
Calc. Lach. Plat. Sil. Sul. Pall.
627.

ailments from egotism. Calc.
Lyc. Sul. Pall. *627*.

FASTIDIOUS.
Ars. Nux. v. *608*.

FORGETFUL.
Pet. *633*. Rhod. *705*. Nux.
mosch. *600*.

FRETFUL.
Puls. *685*.

HAUGHTY.
Plat. Pall. *625*. Caust. Hyos.
Ipec. Lach. Lyc. Plat. Staph.
Stram. Sul. Verat. Pall. *627*.

HYPOCHONDRIAC.
Mez. *551*, Puls. *685*, Anac. *48*,
Con. *321*. Sul. *786*.

IMPATIENT.
Iod. *433*, *434*. Ipec. *444*. Med.
530. Lach. *499*.

HURRIED MANNER.
Ptelea. *679*.

INDECISIVE.
Puls. (Kali sul. *476*).

INDIFFERENT.
Carbo. v. *210*, Con. *321/2* Kali br. *476*, Merc. *544*, Nitric ac. *586*, Picric ac *656*, Plumbum *664*.

INDIFFERENT AND APATHETIC.
Staph. Phos ac. *635 637* Phos. *641*. *644*. Sepia *739*.

INDIFFERENT TO FAMILY.
Sepia *739, 740. 744*. Staph. *761*. Sul. *786*.

INTELLECTUAL.
Lyc. *515*. *520*.

IRRITABLE.
Ferr. *371*. Caust. *222*. Cham. *237*. Cocc. *290*, Cycl. *351*. Cocc. *290*, Ign. *429*. Hepar *405*. Ledum. *507*. Lyc. *516*. Merc. *544*, Mez. *552*. Mur. ac. *566*. Nat. mur. *570*. Nat. sul. *584/5*. Lac. can. *488*, Nitric ac. *586*. *Nux. vom. 602*. Pall *626/7*. Pet. *629*. Psor. *676*. Puls. *685*. Sepia *700*. Tarent. *800*.

JEALOUS.
Lach. Puls. Nux. v. Stram. Hyos. *411/3* Puls. (Kali sul. *476*). Opium. *Lach. 494. 496*.

LACKING GRIT.
Sil. *750*.

LACKING SELF-CONFIDENCE OR SELF-ASSERTION.
Sil. *750*.

LACONIC.
Mur. ac. *566*.

LAZY.
Carbo v. *207*, Caust. *226*. Sul. *786*.

LISTLESS.
Sil. *750*.

LOQUACIOUS.
Dulc. *365*. *Lach. 495/8*. Pyrogen *694*. Hyos (Lach. *496*). *Stram. 769. 771. 776*.

MELANCHOLIC.
Caust. *222*. *226*. Cocc. *290*. Lyc. *516*. Kali carb. *468*. Pet. *632*. Plumbum. *664*. Psor. *676*. Puls. *685*.

as result of history of eruptions. Mez. *556*.

prefers to be alone. Nat. mur. *572*.

MENTAL TRAUMATISM (AN ABNORMAL CONDITION OF BODY CAUSED BY EXTERNAL 'WOUNDS' OF MIND, HEART SOUL).
Plat. *658*. *662*.

NERVOUS.
Caust. *222*. Dros. *362*.

PARANOIAC.
Plat. *658*.

OBSTINATE.
Caps. *205*. Nitric ac. *586*. San. *732*.

PEEVISH.
Alum. *37*. Nux. Bry. Alum. *39*. Aur. *106*. Caust. *222*. *226*. Ant. crud. *53*. Kali carb. *468*. Mur. ac. *564*. Plat. *661*.
'Can't bear it' . . . Cham. *236*.

PUSILLANIMOUS.
Mur. ac. *566*.

QUARRELSOME.
Ran. b. *701*.

RESTLESS.
Phos. *643*. Plat. *601*. Tarent. *798* Pyrogen. *690/2*.

SELFISH.
Med. *530*.

SLOW TO THINK.
Carbo. v. *207*.

SLUGGISH.
Carbo v. *207*, Colch. *308*. Gels. *382*.

STUPID.
Hyos. Bell. (Stram. *771*).

STAMMERING.
Merc. *545*. Stram. *774*. *777*.

FEELING OF SUPERIORITY.
Plat. *658*. *660*.

SUSPICIOUS.
Lach. Puls. Nux. Stram. Hyos. *411/3* Puls. (Kali sul. *476*) Nitric ac. *586*. Lach. Nux. v. Apis *74* Caps. *205*, Caust. *222* Crot. *336*. Cimic. *273*. Dros. *352*. *362*. Merc. *544*.

SUICIDAL.
Cimic. *272*. Alum. *37*. Lil. tig. *508*. Med. *530*. Nat. sul. *584/5 581* Stram. *776*. Psor *674*. Sepia *740, 745* Ornithogalum. *619* Aurum. (Nat. sul. *518*). Ant. crud. *48*.

by drowning only. Dros. *362*

UNCOORDINATED.
Caust. *222*. Ferr. *371*.

UNHAPPY.
Caust. *222*.

YIELDING, GOOD HUMOURED.
Puls. (Kali sul. *476*).

OVERSENSITIVE – See SENSITIVITY.

AILMENTS FROM ENVY AND CHAGRIN.
Staph. *762*, Staph. (Phos. ac. *635*).

EASILY EXCITED TO TEARS AND LAUGHTER.
Puls. (Kali sul. *476*). Lyc. *516*. Nat. mur. *569*.

PROSTRATED, WITH NERVOUS EXHAUSTION.
Cocc. *295*.

EXCESSIVE CONSCIENCE.
Sil. *752*.

TIMID.
Caust. *222*. Kali carb. *468*. Puls. Kali sul. *475*).

MIND CONTINUALLY DWELLING ON SEXUAL MATTERS.
Staph. *767*.

NYMPHOMANIA.
Hyosc. *412*. *Stram. 769. 777* Tarent. *802*.

DESIRE TO UNCOVER.
Hyos. *408*. *413*. Mur. ac. *564*.

due to hyperaesthesia of skin. Hyos. *412*.

EROTOMANIA.
exposing the person. Stram. *772*.

OBSCENE SPEECH.
Stram. *772*.

TEARS CLOTHES OFF HIS BODY.
Ver. alb. *856*. Hyos. *413*.

MANIA WITH LEWDNESS.
Ver. alb. *853*, Hyos. *413*.

LEWDNESS WITH LASCIVIOUS
TALK.
Ver alb. *853*.

LASCIVIOUS.
Hyos. *408, 413*. Ver. alb. *856*.
Tarent. *800*.

DEMENTIA PRAECOX.
Tarent *808*.

IRRESISTIBLE IMPULSE TO KILL.
Plat. *662*.

DELUSIONS OF GRANDEUR.
Ver. alb. *853*.

PAROXYSMS OF TEMPER.
Canth. *196*. Bell. *116*. Cham.
237.

PERSISTENT RAGING.
Var. alb. *853*.

SUDDEN VIOLENT DESTRUCTIVE
MOVEMENTS.
Tarent. *798. 801. 807*. Ver. alb.
856.

SUDDEN IMPULSE TO DO
VIOLENCE.
Hepar *405/6*. Nux. v. *602*.

SADNESS, GRIEF, MORAL
DEPRESSION.
Tarent. *800*.

INTENSELY EMOTIONAL WHILE
INTELLECT IS SLOWED
DOWN.
Plumbum. *665*.

HOPELESSNESS, DESPAIR OF
PERFECT RECOVERY (I.E.
LACK OF VITAL REACTION).
Psor. *672. 674. 676*.

EFFECT OF SHOCK, MENTAL OR
PHYSICAL.
Arn. (Symphitum *793*).

INCLINATION TO DECEIVE AND
FEIGN SICKNESS.
Tarent *800*, Plumbum. *665*.

COMPLAINTS FROM SUPPRESSED
ANGER, OR FEELINGS.
Staph. *761*.

< FROM MENTAL AFFECTIONS,
ANGER WITH INDIGNATION.
Staph. *767*.

< FROM GRIEF.
Staph. *767*.

SUICIDE:
fears of . . . Alum. *36*.
longing for death. Aur. *106.
108. 109*.
in deep depression. Aur. *108*.
feeling of hopelessness Aur.
109.
suicidal feeling. Hepar *406*.
Hyosc. *415*.
loathing of life. Ant. crud. *53*.

PASSIVE MENTAL STATES.
Con. *322*. Ign. *424*.

VIOLENT MENTAL STATES.
Bell. Hyos. Stram. Ars. (Con.
322) Iod. *434*. Nux. v. *602*.

TURMOIL IN THE BRAIN.
Cham. *236*.

ALTERNATE STATES OF
BROODING AND SCREAMING.
Ver. alb. *856*.

'BORDERLINE' INSANITY.
Plat. *658*. Sepia *744*. Lach. *494*.

WARPED MENTALITY.
Staph. *767*.

INSANITY.
Sepia *744*, Tarent. *798. 800*.
Ver. alb. *855*.

< AT NEW MOON.
Sil. *750*.

HYSTERIA, COMPLETE LOSS OF
CONTROL.
Tarent. *798. 800*.

MANIA.
Ver. alb. *856*. Cocc. *290*.
Cimic. *272*. Lach. *499*. *Stram.*
769. Tarent. *801*.

MANIA — PUERPERAL.
Stram. *769*.

HYSTERICAL.
Nux. mosch. *597. 599*. Pall.
626. Plumbum. *665*. Ammon
carb. *46*. Ign. Caul. *219*.
Cimic. *271*.

INABILITY TO THINK.
Med. *530*. Abrot. *1*. Aeth. *19*.
Con. *322*. Hyos. *413*. Gels. *385*.
Sul. ac. *724*.

INABILITY TO FIX ATTENTION.
Aeth. *19*. Ail. *27. 28*. Con. *322*.
327. Lac. can. *488*.

MIND WANDERING.
Nitric ac. *589*. Bapt. *114*.

FORGETFULNESS.
Cann. *180*, Ail. *27*. Anac. *47*.
Nux. mosch. *596. 599*.

MIND GIVES OUT.
Con. *322*.

THOSE WITH A STATE OF
'DISORDER'.
Sul. *783*.

THOSE NOT DISTURBED BY A
STATE OF UNCLEANLINESS.
Sul. *784*.

THE 'RAGGED PHILOSOPHER'.
Sul. *785*.

MENTAL SYMPTOMS DEVELOP
FIRST IN ANY AILMENT.
Phos. ac. *635*.

PHYSICAL SYMPTOMS DEVELOP
FIRST IN ANY AILMENT.
Mur. ac. (Phos. ac. *635*).

VIOLENT CONDUCT.
1. Stram. *2*. Bell. *3*. Hyos.
(more passive) Hyos. *412. 415*.
Abrot. *1*. Aeth. *19*. Bell. *116–
126*.

GLOOM ALTERNATING WITH
PHYSICAL AILMENTS.
Cimic. *276*.

ANXIETY ABOUT OTHERS'
SICKNESS.
Ars. Phos. Sul. Cocc. *290*.

BODY < WHEN MIND IS
CHEERFUL.
Plat. *661*.

BODY > WHEN MIND IS
AFFECTED.
Plat. *661*.

CHRONIC EFFECTS OF GRIEF.
Phos. ac. *636*.

WAKES IN NIGHT THINKING
AWFUL THINGS.
Viscum. *868*.

BREAKDOWN FROM NERVOUS
STRAIN.
Phos. ac. *634*.

DESIRE FOR COMPANY <
ALONE.
Pall. *626*, Phos. *641*.

DESIRE FOR COMPANY >
ALONE.
Sepia. Nat mur. (Phos. *641*).

133

WANTS SYMPATHY.
Phos. *641*.

DISLIKES SYMPATHY.
Nitric ac. *586*. Sepia. Nat.
mur. (Phos. *641*).

FEELS TALL.
Stram Plat. Pall. *625*.

CONDITION RESEMBLES
INTOXICATION.
Stram. *775*.

DRUNKEN CONFUSION.
Nux. v. *603*.

INTOXICATION.
Sul. Camph. Nux. v. *603*.

CONFUSED.
Nux. mosch. *600*.

DAZED, AUTOMATIC
BEHAVIOUR.
Nux. mosch. *600*.

BRAIN FAG.
Picric ac. *656*.

CANNOT ENDURE SLIGHTEST
AILMENT.
Nux. v. *603*.

VEXED AT LEAST TRIFLE.
Nitric ac. *588*, Nux. v. *609*.

EVERY EMOTION ATTENDED
WITH THROBBING.
Kreos. *488*.

LOSS OF SENSE OF TIME.
Lach. *497*. Med. *530*.

LOSS OF LOCATION, FAMILIAR
PLACES LOOK STRANGE.
Opium. Nux. mosch. *596*.
Glon. *389*. Pet. Glon. *393*. Bry.
Opium. *614*.

FIXED IDEAS.
Anac. *49*.

SEARCHES FOR PINS.
Sil. *757*.

DESIRE TO RUN AWAY.
Bell. Mez. *552*.

MENTAL ANGUISH FROM LOSS
OF FRIEND.
Nitric ac. *590*.

ERRORS OF PERCEPTION.
Nux. mosch. *599*.

HYPOCHONDRIAC.
Nux. v. *603*.

LYING AND STEALING.
Opium. *610*.

ARRESTED DEVELOPMENT AS
RESULT OF VACCINATIONS.
Thuja. *827*. *837*.

WANTS TO TRAVEL.
Tub. *835/6*.

WANTS TO BE BUSY.
Ver. alb. *856*.

LOST SENSE OF PROPORTION IN
BOTH OCULAR AND MENTAL
VISION.
Plat. *662*.

BROODS OVER OLD INSULTS
ETC.
Nat. mur. *570*.

MAKES MISTAKES IN WRITING.
Lyc. Lach. *497* Rhod. *705*
Thuja *821*. Alum. *40*. Lyc. *515*.

MAKES MISTAKES IN SPEAKING.
Lil. tig. *509*, Alum. *40*. LYc.
515. Thuja *821*.

IRRESISTIBLE DESIRE TO CURSE.
Anac. *48*. Nat. mur. *571*.

FEELINGS OF WOUNDED PRIDE.
Plat. Pall. *626*.

ALTERNATION OF MENTAL AND
PHYSICAL SYMPTOMS.
Plat. 662.

< NOISE, DARK, BEING ALONE,
EATING, SLEEPING.
Phos. *644.*

IDIOTIC CHILDREN.
Aeth. *17.*

APPEARANCE OF IMBECILITY.
Cocc. *295.* Hyos. *413.*

DELUSIONS OF:
furniture being persons. Nat.
phos. *578.*
footsteps in the next room.
Nat. phos. *578.*
wealth, Pyrogen. *691.*
persecution. Dros. *354.*
being surrounded by
imaginary foes or animals.
Plumbum. *670.* Crot. *336.*
Cycl. *351.*
of many kinds. Hyos. *412.*
Lach. *499.* Opium. *613.*
someone behind. Med. *530.*

INCLINATION TO PRAY.
Stram. *776.*

RELIGIOUS INSANITY.
Lach. *484.* Stram. *776.*
mania. Ver. alb. *856.*

MELANCHOLY.
Psor. *676.*

'FREAKS'.
Puls. *685.*

SPEAKS TO DEAD RELATIONS.
Hyos. *412.*

AILMENTS FROM DISAPPOINTED
LOVE.
Nat. mur. Hyos. Ign. Phos ac.
635.

DISPOSITION TO SILENT
GRIEVING.
Ign. *425.*

CHANGEABLE MOODS.
Ign. *426,* Puls. *686.*

CONTINUED INABILITY TO
CONTROL EMOTIONS.
Nat. mur. (Ign. *427*).

AILMENTS FROM BAD NEWS.
Apis. Calc. Gels. Ign. Med.
Nat. mur. Sul. Pall. *627.*

AILMENTS RESULTING FROM
INSULTS AND GRIEVANCES.
Staph. Acon. *4.*

EASILY EXCITED, WITH
INCREDIBLY RAPID CHANGES
OF MOOD.
Ign. (Phos. ac. *635*).

INCLINATION TO LAUGH AT
EVERYTHING.
Nux. mosch. *586.*

INVOLUNTARY LAUGHTER AND
TEARS.
Puls. (Kali sul. *476*).

TENDENCY TO INWARD GRIEF
AND PEEVISHNESS.
Puls. *681.*

OVERWROUGHT, INTENSE.
Ign. *427.* Mur. ac. *590.*

MILD, TIMID, YIELDING,
LACHRYMOSE DISPOSITION.
Puls. *681.*

SLOW, PHLEGMATIC
TEMPERAMENTS.
Puls. *681*.

TREMBLING ANXIETY. >
MOTION.
Puls. *685*.

CHILD CRIES PITIFULLY.
Puls. *686*.

CHILD CRIES IN SNARLING
MANNER.
Cham. (Puls. *686*).

SUDDEN CHANGES OF MOOD.
Crocus. Tarent. *798*.

EXTREME DISPOSITION TO
LAUGH AND JOKE.
Tarent. *800*.

MANIA TO KISS EVERYBODY.
Crocus. Ver. alb. *856*.

WEEPS WITH JOY.
Lyc. *522*.

SENTIMENTAL AND EMOTIONAL.
Nat. mur. *570*.

DOES NOT WANT TO BE
TOUCHED.
Ant. crud. Cham. San. *732*.

CANNOT BEAR TO BE TOUCHED
OR LOOKED AT
(SCOPOPHOBIA).
Ant. crud. *52*. Kali carb. *473*.

SUDDEN CHANGES OF HUMOUR.
Cycl. *351*. Ign. *429*. Puls. (Kali
sul. *476*). Nat. mur. *571*.

WANTS SOMEONE NEAR ALL
THE TIME.
Dros. *362*. Lyc. *514*.

IMAGINES EVERYTHING LOOKS
SMALL.
Plat. *662*. Cop. Stram. (Pall.
625).

IMAGINES SHE IS TWO PEOPLE.
Bapt. Pet. Pyrogenium. Nux.
mosch. *595/6*.

HALLUCINATIONS.
Rhus. *712*, Kali br. *467*. Med.
530. Merc. *544*. Opium. *616*.

CONSTANT IRRESISTIBLE
DESIRE TO LOOK BEHIND.
Brom. Lach. Med. San. *733*.

INVOLUNTARY MOVEMENTS
WHILE AWAKE. > ASLEEP.
Agar. *26*.

FITS OF UNCONTROLLABLE
WEEPING.
Kali br. *466*, Lil. tig. *512*. Lyc.
516.

RAPID ALTERNATIONS OF
GAIETY AND DISPOSITION TO
WEEP.
Ign. *424*. *429*. Nux. mosch.
599.

DISLIKES BEING SPOKEN TO.
Hyos. *413*. Puls. (Kali sul
476). Nat. sul. *584*.

WANTS TO GO HOME.
Bry. Hyos. *413*.

THOSE WHO KEEP THEIR
ANNOYANCE TO
THEMSELVES.
Ign. *424*.

ANGER, EAGERNESS AND
VIOLENCE PREDOMINATING.
Nux. (Ign. *424*). Lac. can. *488*.
Nux. v. *602*.

WANTS SOMETHING THEN
THROWS IT AWAY.
Cham. Kreos *484*. Cina.
Staph. *764 766*.

TEMPER OVER IMAGINARY
INSULTS.
Staph. Cham. *237*.

TEMPER OVER UNIMPORTANT
CIRCUMSTANCES.
Dros. *362*

STRAIN FROM OVERWORK.
Arn. (China *257*).

MERCURY POISONING.
Mur.ac. *563*, Nitric ac. *588*.

METEORISM
DISTENSION OF ABDOMEN BY
GAS PRODUCED IN
INTESTINES.
see ABDOMEN and
VETERINARY.

METRITIS
INFLAMMATION OF THE WOMB.
see FEMALE SEX.

METRORRHAGIA
BLEEDING FROM WOMB AT
TIMES OTHER THAN DURING
MENSES.
see FEMALE SEX.

MIASMS
Tub. *840*.

MIGRAINE
PAROXYSMAL HEADACHES.
Cann. *179*.

WITH VOMITING.
Cocc. 291

MODALITIES
INTENSE DREAD OF
DOWNward MOTION.
Borax. 132. 135. Gels. San. *737*.

STAGGERING WHEN GETTING
UP FROM SITTING.
Calc. p. *167*

SEASICKNESS.
Cocc. *297*, Glon. *390*. Pet. *630*.
633.

MOTION BRINGS ON PAINFUL
SENSATION AS OF ELECTRIC
VIBRATION.
Colch. *306*.

SPASM FROM JAR.
Nux. v. Strych. Bell. Cicuta
264.

FROM:
upward or downward motion.
Borax. *134*.

laying children down in bed.
Borax. *134, 137*.

going upstairs. Calc. p. *166*.

bending forward. Chel. *248*.

rapid motion. Ferr. *372*.

on walking. Ars. (Gels. 384).

at rest. Rhus. *707*.
Taraxacum. (Rhus *707*) Ferr.
372. Rhus. Nat. sul. *582*.

< heat of bed. *Merc. 537*. Led.
Mer. *539*.

while sweating. Merc. *537*.

washing. Sul. Ammon. carb.
43.

pressure. *Bell. 123*. Chel. *248*.
(Bry. *144*).

jar. Ferr. phos. *379*.

Theridion. *817*. Cocc. *291*.
Bell. *117, 119, 123*. Cicuta *264*.
Chel. *248*.

sitting up Cocc. *293*.
moving Cocc. *293*. Pet. *629/
630*. Rhus. Pyrogen. *690*. Bell.
119. 123. 125 Bry. *143. 152*.
Chel. *248*. Colch. *303. 306*.
Bry. (Gels. *384*) Nat. sul. *582*.

moving, but > for continued
motion. Rhus. (Pyrogen *690*)
Rhus. 709.

riding in a carriage or boat.
Cocc. 293, Pet. *629. 630*.

smoking. Cocc. *293*.

talking. Cocc. *293, 298*.

eating. Cocc. *293. 298*.

drinking. Cocc. *293. 298*.

night watching. Cocc. *293 298*.

loss of sleep Cocc. *293, 298*,
Lach. Crot. *(335)*.

on waking. Lach. Crot. *(335)*.

lying on painful side. Ruta.
719.

anger. Ign. *425*.

mental exertion. Ign. *425*.

strong smells. Ign. *425*.

when yawning. Ign. *425*.

kneeling. Sepia. (Nitric ac.
587).

study. Picric ac. *656*.

movement of eyes. Picric ac.
656.

looking fixedly at an object.
Ruta. *719*.

eating uncooked food Ruta.
719.

least touch. *Staph. 767*.

noise. *Theridion. 816*. Borax.
133. Ferr. *373*.

closing eyes. Theridion. *807*.

light. Theridion. *817*. Bell *117.
119. 120/1*.

anxiety. Cocc. *293*. Ign. *425*.

lying down. Brom. *138*. Calc.
159.

> FROM:

seeing moving objects. Cocc.
295.

at rest. Bry. (Rhus. *707*).

slow gentle motion. Ferr. *372*.
Puls (Ferr. *373*).

at seaside. *Med. 529*. Nat. mur.
568.

heat of bed. Ars. (Merc. *539*).

rolling from side to side.
Tarent. *802*.

pressure. *Bry. 144*. China. *258*,
Cimic. *271*.

moving. Puls. *682*. Brom. *138*.
Cimic. *271*. Ferr. *372*. Rhus
Ruta *719*.

lying quiet. Cocc. *293*.

lying on painful side. Ign. *425*.
Bry. (Ptelea *680*) Pyrogen *691,
695*.

lying on right side. Phos. *646,
Merc. 537*.

bending limbs. Cocc. *294*.

letting limbs hang down. Con.
323.

being rubbed. Phos. *642*.

binding head tightly. Picric
ac. *656*.

138

slow movement. Ferr. Puls.
681.

music. *Tarent 798, 780*.

for milk. Chel. *249*.

EXERTION CAUSES FAINTNESS.
Ferr. 372.

MORBUS BASEDOWII
BASEDOW'S DISEASE.
see GOITRE.

MORBUS BRIGHTII
BRIGHT'S DISEASE.
see KIDNEYS.

MOUTH
TASTE – foul, like putrid water.
Caps. *200*.

strong, metallic. Cocc. Merc.
Nat. c. Rhus. Senega. (Cup
342). Cocc. *296*. Merc. *538*.

burnt. Puls. *684*.

bitter. Nux. v. *605*, Stram. *777*,
Cycl. *351*, Bry. *149*. Calc. p.
168. Chel. *247. 250*. Ferr. *372*.

putrid. Puls. *684*. Pyrogen *694*.
Cycl. *351*.

putrid on coughing. Nux. v.
605.

salty. Theridion. *816*. Merc.
540, 542. Cycl. *351*.

tasteless. Ver. alb. *854*.

unbearable. Ferr. *372*.

mouldy. Ledum. *507*.

of rotten eggs. Merc. *540, 542*.
Ferr. *372*.

slimy. Merc. *540 542*.

sweet. Merc. *540, 542*.

coppery. Cimic *273*. Med. *531*.

fatty, rancid. Asaf. *103*.

flat, offensive. Anac. *48*. Bry.
149. Cycl. *351*.

> cold water. Bry. *159*.

COLD.
Carbo v. 211.

DRY.
Kali bich. *458*. Nux mosch.
599. Sal. ac. *724*, Ver. vir. *861*,
Acon. *9*. Ant. crud. *55*. Ars. *99*.
Bapt. *113/4* Bry. *148* Cann.
182. Caps. *200* Glon. *394*.

DRY,
but seldom thirsty. Puls. *686*.

DRY,
with great thirst. Rhus. *711*.

BLEEDING.
Bapt. *112*.

SWOLLEN.
Bapt. *113*.

BURNING.
Tereb. *810*. Caps. *199, 200*.
Iris. *450*. Mez. *552*. Phos. *643*.
honey-like scabs around.
Mex. 553

APHTHOUS.
Nitric ac. *591*, Sul. 788

ULCERATED.
Bapt. *113. 115*. Calc. *160*.
Merc. *541/2* Phyt. *652*. Mur.
ac. *564* Nitric ac. *590*.

ULCERATED.
feeling of splinters in mouth
Nitric ac. *593*.

CANCRUM ORIS
(gangrenous ulcer) Caps. 203.

YELLOW CREAMY COATING ON
BACK PART OF ROOF OF
MOUTH.
Nat. phos. 576.

SMELL FROM MOUTH FOUL,
cadaverous. Nitric ac. 590.

JAWS AS IF PARALYSED.
Nux. mosch. 597.

ACCUMULATION OF WATER
IN . . .
Pet. 632/3

CANKER SORES.
SAL. AC. 724.

INFLAMMATION OF SALIVARY
GLANDS.
Sil. 753.

WITH SORE CORNERS.
Ant. crud. 52, Graph. 395.

CRACKS IN CORNERS OF . . .
Ant. crud. 53. 55.

ERUPTIONS AROUND . . .
Ars. 100.

FOAMING HAVING ODOUR OF
EGGS.
Bell. 124.

> IF MOISTENED.
BRy. Borax. 133.

BLISTERS.
Caps. 200, Med. 534.

WHITE AND BLUE ROUND . . .
Cina. 282.

ERUPTIONS IN CORNER OF . . .
Graph. 400.

SYPHILITIC AFFECTIONS.
Kali bich. 458.

HAWKING TENACIOUS MUCOUS.
Kali bich. 458.

EXPECTORATION, SALTY.
Phos. Ars. Sepia.Lyc . . Puls.
Phos ac. 636.

FAUCES:
deepseated ulcers of . . . Kali
bich. 458

dark red. Bapt. 115.

dry. Bell. 122. 124.

spasms of . . . Bell. 122.

MUCOUS IN MOUTH.
Chel. 250.

STOMATITIS.
Sal. ac. 724. Merc. 545.

PALATE:
raw. Ant. crud. 55, Bapt. 113.
San. 733. Stram. 771.

dark red. Bell. 122.

membrane seems burnt.
Borax. 137.

syphilitic ulcers in . . . Aur.
110.

BREATH:
fetid. Plumbum. 668, Ail. 28.
Sal. ac. 724. Acon. 10 Merc.
Bapt. 115. Cham. 239. Kreos.
478.

very offensive as in phthisis
Psos. 674.

foul and offensive. Merc. 537.
545.

putrid odour. Kreos 478/9.
Cham. 239. Merc. Bapt. 115.

GUMS:
mercurio-syphilitic disease
of . . . Hepar. 406.

pale. Med. *534*. Plumbum. *668*.

swollen. Merc. *542*. Plumbum. *668*. Caust. *227*.

spongy. Merc. *545*.

bleeding. Merc. *545*. Phos. ac. *637*. Sal. ac. *726*. Staph. *762* Ars. *94*. Carbo v. *212*. Hepar. *406*.

ulcerated. Merc. *545*.

burning. Tereb. *810*.

blue, purple or brown. Plumbum. *668*.

bluish, red, soft, spongy, easily bleeding, inflamed, ulcerated.

scorbutic. Merc. *542*. Kreos. *479*. *482*.

painful. Plumbum. *668*. Kreos. *482*.

abscesses of . . . Caust. *227*.

SALIVA:

offensive. Merc. Nitric ac. *588*.

fetid, acrid, bloody. Nitric ac. *591*.

dribbling. Stram. *774*.

saltish. Ant. crud. *55*.

white, thick, frothy. Cann. *182*.

profuse. Ipec. *444*. Iod. *432*. Iris. *450*, Ledum. *505*. Merc. *538/9* Nitric ac. *591*

MUCOUS MEMBRANES

DRY AND IRRITATED.
Alum. *35*.

BURNING. Caps. *199*, Kreos *483*.

RAW.
Kreos. *484*.

SLIMY.
Merc. *537*.

PALE.
Phos. *646*.

DISEASES OF MUCOUS MEMBRANES ANYWHERE.
Kali bich. *454*. Sal. ac. *725*.

GENERALLY AFFECTED.
Ant. crud. *54*, Kreos. *478*.

DEGENERATION.
Mez. 556.

ULCERATION OF.
Kreos. *482*. Mur. ac. *563*. Arg. nit. *78*.

HYPERAEMIA OF ALIMENTARY CANAL.
Canth. *194*.

INFLAMMATION OF:
alimentary tract. Canth . . . *195*.

genito-urinary. Canth. *194*.

respiratory tract. Ant. tart. *67*.

CATARRHAL INFLAMMATIONS.
Ant. tart. *68*.

SLOW INTENSE INFLAMMATIONS.
Kali bich. *455*.

HAEMORRHAGES OF.
Phos. Ars. *95*, Sal. ac. *725*.

WITH THICK YELLOW OFFENSIVE MUCOUS.
Cistus *287*. Kali bich. *455*.

PSEUDO-MEMBRANOUS
FORMATIONS ON . . .
Chlorine, Bromine, Iod. *435*.

DISCHARGES ROPY AND
STRINGY.
Kali bich. *453, 455, 458/9*.

MEMBRANES OF THROAT
GLISTENING.
Lac. can. *491*.

TWITCHING OF MUSCLES OF
CHEEK.
Mez. *546*.

CONDYLOMATA.
Nitric ac. *592/3* Staph. *767*.
Thuja *828*.

PURPURA HAEMORRHAGICA.
Sal. ac. *725*.

MUMPS
Pilocarpine. Carbo veg. *211*.

MUSCLES
TWITCHING.
Agar. *26* Caust. *223*, Mez. *546*.
Tarent. *798*.

CLUMSY, DROPS THINGS.
Agar *22*.

SOFT AND FLABBY.
Ammon. carb. *44*.

CONTRACTIONS.
Caust. *223*.

CONTRACTIONS (TORTICOLLIS)
Caust. *224*

EXCESSIVE SORENESS AND
JERKING.
Cimic. *272, 276*.

PAINS IN MUSCLES < COLD
DAMP WEATHER.
Phyt *651*.

FEEL BRUISED AND SORE TO
TOUCH.
Acon. Arn. Bry. Ran. b. *702*
Ruta 718.

MYALGIA (MUSCLE PAIN)
Arn. *90*. Cimic *271, 274*.

DIFFICULTY IN CO-ORDINATION.
Agar. *22*. Cimic. *276*.

WEAKNESS OF CERVICAL
MUSCLES.
Opium. *615*.

PROGRESSIVE MUSCULAR
ATROPHY. PLUMBUM. *665/6*.

FIBRILLARY CONTRACTION
IN . . .
Plumbum. *666*.

MUSCULAR ATROPHY FROM
SCLEROSIS OF SPINAL
SYSTEM.
Plumbum. *669*.

RHEUMATISM OF . . .
Ran. b. *699*.

INTERCOSTAL RHEUMATISM.
Ran. b. 701;

LOSS OF POWER.
Ruta *718*.

MYOSITIS OSSIFICANS.
Thuja. *820*.

FORMICATION OF GLUTEAL
MUSCLES.
Agar. *25*.

MYALGIA
MUSCLE PAIN. See MUSCLES.

MYOMA UTERIS
See UTERUS.

MYOSOTIS
inflammation of muscles.
see MUSCLES.

NATES
BUTTOCKS.
Graph. *400*.

NAUSEA
Acon. *9*. Ail. *28*. Allium. *32*.
Ant. crud. *52*. Cocc. *293*.
Colch. *302*.

WITH:
pale face. skin cool, moist and
relaxed. Ant. tart. *60*.

feeble pulse. Ant. tart. *60*.

muscular relaxation. Ant.
tart. *60*.

gastric unease. Ant. tart. *60*.

saliva flowing copiously Ant.
tart. *60*.

great faintness. Ant. tart. *66*,
Borax. *136*. Sepia *741*.

dilated pupils. Cimic. *272*.
Glon. *393*.

pain in stomach. Collin *311*.
Ipec. *445*.

chronic constipation. Collin.
311.

asthma. Ipec. *439*. *440*.

all complaints. *Ipec. 441 445*.

burning pain in arms. Kali
bich. *460*.

pallor, cold sweat. Pet. *631*.

ALL DAY.
Pet. *633*.

CONSTANT.
Ptelea *680*. Ant. tart. *65/7*. *Arg.
nit. 80*. Nat. sul. *582*. Ipec. *437*.

INTENSE.
Ipec. Ant. tart. *63*

IN HEPATITIS.
Chel. *250*.

AT WORK.
Borax. *136*.

FELT IN HEAD.
Cocc. *298*.

FELT IN RECTUM.
Ruta *719*.

CEREBRAL.
Glon. *393*.

IN ABDOMEN.
Puls. Ruta *719*.

IN STOMACH.
Ipec. Ruta. *719*.

IN THROAT.
Cycl. Phos.ac. Stann. Ruta
719.

WHEN RIDING IN A CARRIAGE.
Sepia *741*.

FROM SMOKING.
Calc. p. *168*.

FROM COFFEE.
Calc. p. *168*.

DURING GESTATION.   Collin.
311.

NOT RELIEVED BY VOMITING.
Ipec. *437*.

DESIRE TO COUGH AND VOMIT
SIMULTANEOUSLY.
Ipec. *437, 439, 440*.

MORNINGS ONLY.
Sepia *741*.

RESULT OF SIGHT, SMELL OR THOUGHT OF FOOD.
Sepia *741*, Ars. Sep. Cocc. Colch. *303*.

AFTER A MEAL.
Ammon carb. *42*. Nux. v. *605*.

ON CLOSING EYES.
Theridion. *815*.

< SLIGHTEST MOTION.
Theridion. *815*.

> WALKING.
Ptelea *680*.

< WARMTH.
Tabac (Pet *631*).

> IN OPEN AIR.
Tabac. (Pet *631*).

> AFTER VOMITING.
Ant. tart. *63*.

> AFTER EATING.
Sepia *741*.

IN VOMITING OF PREGNANCY.
Chel. *250*. Ipec. *437*.

N

NECK
STIFF.
Sil. *753*. Calc. *162*, Calc. p. *166*. Caust. *228* Cicuta *264* Cimic. *271/2*.

RIGID.
Calc. *162*. Calc. p. *166*. Chel. *251*

WITH PAIN IN OCCIPUT.
Caust. *228*.

TENSION OR CRAMP.
Cicuta *263*.

RETRACTED.
Cimic. *272*.

RHEUMATIC PAINS.
Cimic. *272*.

TORTICOLLIS (CONTRACTION OF FLEXOR TENDONS).
Cimic *274*. Caust *224*. *230*.

GLANDS ENLARGED AND KNOTTED.
Cistus *288* (as in Hodgkin's disease).

STIFF AS RESULT OF COLD.
Dulc. *365*.

STIFF AS RESULT OF SITTING IN DRAUGHT.
Rhus. *710*.

NECROSIS
DEATH OF TISSUE OF BONE. see BONES.

NEONATORIUM
OF FIRST YEAR OF LIFE.
Nitric ac. *590*

NEPHRITIS
INFLAMMATION OF KIDNEYS.
Canth. *194*. Kali carb. *471*, see KIDNEYS

NERVES
INJURIES TO.
Hyp. 416, 418, 423.

INJURIES TO PARTS RICH IN
NERVES.
Hyp. *416* (Ledum. *503*).

SHOOTING PAINS, SCIATICA.
Hyp. *419*.

EFFECTS OF NERVOUS SHOCK.
Hyp. 423.

PAINS IN NERVE TISSUES.
Mag. phos. *527*.

NEURASTHENIA.
Phos ac. *638*.

NEURITIS
inflammation of . . .
Hyp. *418*.
in amputated stump. Allium.
31.
in face. Ars. *95*.

TERRIBLE PAIN.
Mag. phos. Spig. Coloc.
(Ferr. phos. *377*).

NEURALGIA
NERVE PAIN

STARTING AT OCCIPUT AND
OVER VERTEX.
Caust. *229*, Chel. *249*.

RIGHT SUPRA ORBITAL.
Chel. *249*.

FACIAL.
Mez. *555*.

FACIAL. < EATING.
Mez. *555*.

FACIAL. > RADIANT HEAT.
Mez. *555*.

TEETH.
Mez. *555*.

SHIN BONE.
Mez. *555*.

CILIARY, BEFORE STORM.
Rhod. *705*.

OVER RIGHT EYE.
Sang. *729*. Thuja. *823*.

CHRONIC.
Vib. *863*.

AS THOUGH ICE TOUCHED THE
PARTS.
Agar. *25*.

AS THOUGH HOT NEEDLES
TOUCHED THE PARTS.
Ars. Agar. *25*.

INTERCOSTAL FOLLOWING
HERPES ZOSTER.
Ran. b. *699*, Ars. Mez. *554*,
555.

< IN BAD WEATHER.
Rhod. *705*.

> BY WARMTH.
Mag. phos. *525, 527*.

> BY PRESSURE.
Mag. phos. *527*.

FOLLOWED BY MANIA.
Cimic *272*.

SEVERE TEARING PAINS.
Coloc *315*. Ruta. *720*.

EXCRUCIATING.
Mag. phos. *524*.

DAILY AT SAME HOUR.
Kali bich. *458*.

RESULT OF ANGER WITH
INDIGNATION.
Coloc. *315*.

NEURASTHENIA
NERVOUS EXHAUSTION. see
NERVES.

NOSE

RED.
Alum. *36*. Merc. *540*.

TIP SHINY RED.
Borax. *136*. Caps. *202, 204*.

HARD AND RED.
Kali carb. *472*.

OBSTRUCTED.
Ammon. carb. *45*. Calc. *160*.
Kali bich. *457*.

STUFFED UP.
Kali bich. *457*. Lyc. *517*.

VERY DRY.
Kali bich. *457*. NOT merc.
(Merc. *540*).

BLEEDING.
Caust. *227*. Crot. *335*. Ferr.
371. Med. *531*. Pet. *633*.

ITCHING.
Cina *280. 282*. Nitric ac. *590*.
Theridion. *816*.

BURNING IN . . .
Cistus. *287*.

SWELLING AND INFLAMMATION.
Sul. *787*.

TICKLING IN . . .
Caps. *201*.

FISSURES IN . . .
Caust. *224*.

NUMBNESS.
Asaf. *105*.

ULCERATION.
Aur. *109, 110* Kali bich. *457*.
Sul. Merc. *538*. Nitric ac. *590*
Puls. *684*.

SORE NOSTRILS.
Ant. crud. *52*. Aur. *110*. Calc.
160. Med. *531*. Merc. *538*.

PAINFUL.
Ant. crud. *55*. Coloc. *318*.
Graph. *399*.

COLD.
Arn. *85*. Camph. *176*. Carbo v.
207. 211. Cistus. *287*.

**PAINFUL DOWNWARD
PRESSURE.**
Borax. *136*.

MUCH SNEEZING.
Sal. ac. *724*. Sul. *797*.
Theridion. *816*.

ERUPTIONS ON . . .
Mez. *555*

OZAENA – POLYPS.
Asaf. *113*. Kali bich. *456*.
Nitric ac. *590*. Allium *31* Calc.
160. Calc. p. *167*. Sang. *729*.
Sepia *740*.
with coryza. Theridion. *816*.

**FAN-LIKE MOTION OF ALAE
NASI.**
Ant. tart. Bapt. Bell. Brom.
Hell. Lyc. Phos. Rhus.
Pyrogen. *690* Lyc *517. 519*.

DISCHARGING.
nostrils, red. Ars. *93, 98*. Mez.
553.
offensive. Asaf. *102/3. 105. Aur.*
109.
green. Kali bich. *457*. Puls.
Kali sul. *475* Nat. sul. 584.
yellow. Kali bich. *453*. Puls.
Kali sul. 475.

146

WITH PLUG IN NOSTRILS.
Kali bich. *457.*

WITH CLINKERS IN NOSTRILS.
Kali bich. *457.*

AS IF NOSE WOULD BURST.
Kali bich. *459.* Asaf. *103.*

FEELS HEAVY.
Kali bich. *457.*

SEPTUM ULCERATED.
Kali bich. *457.*

SMELL ABNORMALLY ACUTE.
Graph *399.*

FLUIDS ESCAPE THROUGH
NOSE.
Gels. Hyos. *412.*

PRESSURE ON ROOT OF . . .
Hyos. *413.*

MUCOUS TOUGH, ROPY.
Kali bich. *457.*

FETID SMELL FROM NOSE.
Kali bich. *457.* Merc. *451.*

AS IF HAIR IN NOSTRIL.
Kali bich. *549.*

HAEMORRHAGES IN . . .
Ledum. *504*, Sal. ac. *726.*

FOOD AND DRINK
REGURGITATING THROUGH
NOSE.
Gels. Diph. Lyc. *517.*

VIOLENT SNEEZING.
Opium. *615.*

LUPUS ON . . .
Kreos *478.*

CARIES OF BONE.
Asaf. *102.* Aur. *109.*

SORE NASAL BONES.
Aur. *110.* Merc. *541.*

LARGE PEDUNCULATED NASAL
POLYPI.
Calc. p. *167/8.*

PIMPLES, ULCERS, CRUSTS ON
TIP OF NOSE.
Caust. *227.*

WARTS.
Caust. *227.*

SENSATION THAT EVERY
INSPIRATION BRINGS COLD
AIR INTO BRAIN.
Cimic. *275.*

BORING AND PICKING AT . . .
Cina *281., 284.* Arum. tryph.
(Cina *281*).

EPITHELIOMA.
Con. 323.

< WARM ROOM.
Kali sul. *476.*

NOSODE THEORY.
Morb. *558–560.* Tub. *830.*

NUN'S MURMUR IN VEINS.
Ferr. *371.*

NYCTALOPIA
NIGHT BLINDNESS. see EYES.

NYSTAGMUS.
INVOLUNTARY JERKY
MOVEMENTS OF EYES. see
EYES.

O

OBESITY

TENDENCY TO.
Calc. *156*. Caps. *201*. Graph.
Ferr. *374*.

DUE TO IMPROPER NUTRITION.
Calc. Graph. *396*.

ODONTALGIA

TOOTHACHE. see TEETH.

OESOPHAGUS.

PAIN IN STOMACH EXTENDING
TO . . .
Aeth. *20*, Cimic, *275*.

VIOLENT PRESSIVE PAIN IN . . .
Alum. *34*.

SPASMODIC PRESSIVE PAIN
IN . . .
Alum. *34*. Asaf. *103*. Crot. *336*.

RAW, BURNING AFTER A MEAL.
Ammon. carb. *42*.

DRY.
Cocc. *296*.

BURNING IN . . .
Sang. *729*.

SENSATION OF LUMP IN . . .
San. *735*.

FORMICATION IN . . .
Ign. *430*.

GURGLING IN . . . WHEN
SWALLOWING.
Cup. *344*.

PARALYSIS OF . . .
Caust. *223/4*. Gels. *382*. Hyos.
412.

CONTRACTION.
Alum. *34*. *37*.

SENSE OF CONSTRICTION.
Alum. *37*. Bapt. *115*. Cicuta
262.

SENSATION OF BALL RISING
FROM STOMACH.
Asaf. *102*. Con. *323*.

INABILITY TO SWALLOW.
Cicuta. *262*. *265*. Gels. *382*.

PARESIS, EXTENDING TO
PARALYSIS.
Con. *323*.

DIFFICULTY IN GETTING FOOD
PAST CARDIAC ORIFICE.
Con. *323*.

PULSATION IN STOMACH AND
THROUGH . . .
Ferr. *372*.

FOOD DESCENDS SLOWLY.
Kali carb. *472*.

DEGENERATION OF MUCOUS
MEMBRANES.
Kreos *478*.

ONANISM

MASTURBATION.
Ferr. *371*. Phos. ac. *638*.
Tarent. *802*.

ONYCHIA

INFLAMMATION AFFECTING THE
NAILS. see NAILS.

OOPHORITIS

OVARITIS OR INFLAMMATION OF
OVARIES.
Pall. *627*.

OPISTHOTONOS

BENDING BACKWARDS OF HEAD, NECK AND SPINE. see SPINE & CONVULSIONS.

OPHTHALMIA

INFLAMMATION OF EYE. see EYES.

ORTHOPNEA

SEROUS AFFECTIONS OF HEART AND LUNG, DIFFICULTY IN BREATHING IN. see CHEST.

ORGAN DISEASES.
Bellis *131*.

ORGANOPATHY. ORGANOTHERAPY

TREATMENT OF DISEASE BY ADMINISTRATION OF ANIMAL PRODUCTS.
Cean. *231*.

OS (uteri)
ORIFICE OF THE UTERUS.
Caul. *216*. Bell. *124*.

OTALGIA
EARACHE. see EARS.

OTORRHEA
DISCHARGE FROM THE EARS. see EARS.

OYSTER SHELL
Calc. *153*. *158*.

OZAENA

FETID POLYP IN NOSE. see NOSE.

P

PAGET'S DISEASE
Dros. Asaf. *104*.

PAIN
VIOLENT.
Aeth. *19*. Mez. *546*.
VIOLENTLY BURNING.
Caps. Merc. *546*. Tarent *805*.
INTOLERABLE.
Acon. *9*. Cham. *236*.
BURNING
Tereb. *810*. Canth. *196*. Tarent *805*.
BORING.
Asaf. *110*.
STITCHING AND STICKING.
Bry. *144*. Hepar. Nit.ac. (Calc. s. *172*).
CUTTING.
Bell. *125*. Kali carb. *469*.
TEARING.
Bell. *125*. Cham. *237*.
INSUPPORTABLE, DRIVING TO DESPAIR.
Coffea. *300*.
STITCHING.
Kali carb. *469*. Thuja *829*.
FROM PUNCTURED WOUNDS.
Ledum. *500–507*.

SENSATION OF.
Bell. *117.*

SUDDEN.
Bell. *118/9.*

RUNNING ALONG LIMBS.
Bell. *125.*

INTENSE AND RAPID.
Canth. *195.*

INTERMITTENT.
Caul *217.*

SHORT AND CRAMPY.
Caul *217.*

'OUT OF PROPORTION'
Cham. *237.*

  cf. 'prostration out of
proportion' Ars. (Cham. *237*).

OVERSENSITIVE TO.
Acon. Cham. Coffea, Ign. *426.*

RADIATE FROM A CENTRE.
Berberis (Kali bich. *453*).

APPEAR IN SPOTS.
Kali bich. *453. 458.*

APPEAR RAPIDLY AND
DISAPPEAR RAPIDLY.
Kali bich. *458.*

ON UNCOVERED PARTS.
Kali carb. *469.*

NOT FOR PEOPLE WHO ARE
CALM AND PATIENT.
Cham. *236.*

FROM BLUNT INSTRUMENTS.
Arn. *85.*

FROM SURGICAL OPERATIONS.
Arn. *85.*

FROM EXERTION.
Arn. 90.

BURNING PAINS > HEAT.
Ars. *94*, Kali carb. *469.*

NON-BURNING PAINS > HEAT.
Mag. phos. *526.*

NON-BURNING PAINS > COLD.
Phos. *642.* Sal. ac. *725.*

SLIGHTEST PAIN RESULTS IN
EXCESSIVE SINKING OF
STRENGTH.
Ars. *100.*

LOCALLY IN NERVE,
INCREASING IN INTENSITY.
Mag. phos. *527.*

WITH:

  irritability. Cham. *236.* Acon.
6. Colch. *309.*

  excitement. Coffea (Acon. *6*)
Canth. *195.*

  fear. Acon. *6.*

  numbness. Plat. Cocc. Cham.
237.

  sensation of crawling,
numbness, coldness. Calc. p.
166.

  thirst and burning. Apis *72.*

IN:

  cheeks. Acon. *9.*

  chest. Acon. *10. 11.*

  lower lumbar vertebrae.
Acon. 10. Aesc. *13.*

  heart and chest. Acon. *6.*

  head. Bell. Acon. *6.*

  sacro-ileac area. Aesc. *12.*

  rectum. Nit. ac. Aesc. *12. 13.*

  back of neck. Ail. *28/9.*

  upper part of back. Ail. *28.*

  right hip joint. Ail. *28.*

PINCHING SQUEEZING.
Phos ac. *635*

LIKE ELECTRIC SHOCKS.
Phyt. *651*

LIKE SPLINTERS, STITCHING.
Sil. *752.*

CRAMPING PAINS, DEVELOPING
INTO CONVULSIONS.
Plat. *662.*

VERY SENSITIVE TO TOUCH.
Ledum. *500.*

INTERMITTENT OR SPASMODIC.
Mag. phos. *524.*

TERRIBLE, EXCRUCIATING.
VIOLENT.
Mag. phos. *526.* Ver. alb. *857.*

SPLINTER LIKE (ON
MOVEMENT)
Nitric ac. 587.

STINGING IN.
Apis. Merc. *539.* Thuja. *829.*

LIKE KNIVES. ACON. *5.*

VERY FINE, STINGING,
BURNING.
Acon. *11.* Apis. *72.*

LIKE BEESTINGS.
Apis. *72.*

AS IF BRUISED.
Arn. 90.

< during rest. Kali carb. *469.*
474.

< from cold. Kali carb. *469.*
Mag. phos. *527.* Ruta. *720.*

< pressure. Kali carb. *469/470*
474.

< lying on affected side. Kali
carb. *469, 474.*

> during rest. Bry. (Kali
carb. *469, 474*).

< slightest movement. Bry
(Kali carb. *469*) Acon. *9.* Phyt.
651. Colch. *309.*

> pressure. Bry. (Kali carb.
469) Mag. phos. *527.*

> lying on affected side. Bry.
(Kali carb. *469*).

< heat. Bry. (Kali carb *469*).

< touch. Kali carb. *470.*
Staph. *765.*

> cold. Ledum. *500.*

< at night. Mez. *546.* Phyt.
651.

< movement. SI1. *754.*

< lying down. Ruta *720.*

< during stool. Nit.ac. Aesc.
14.

< inhaled cold air. Aesc. *15.*

<noise. Coffea (Acon. *6*).
Canth. *195.*

TO ABOLISH PAIN.
Ars. (Opium *611*).

PAIN FROM INCREASED
SENSITIVITY.
Opium. *611.*

PAINLESSNESS FROM NORMAL
AILMENTS.
Opium. *611. 616.* Stram *771.*

CROSSING FROM SIDE TO SIDE.
Ant. crud. *52.*

CROSSING FROM LEFT TO
RIGHT.
Lach. (Ant. crud. *52*).

151

CROSSING FROM RIGHT TO LEFT.
Lyc. (Ant. crud. *52*).

CROSSING FROM ONE SIDE TO ANOTHER AND BACK.
Lac. can. (Ant. crud. *52*) *Lac. can.* 487, 489.

MOVING FROM ONE PART TO ANOTHER.
Kali bich. *458. 461.*

PALPITATIONS
Acon. *9.*

VIOLENT IN HEART. AETH. *20.*

WITH NAUSEA, HEADACHE
Brom. *140.*

WITH NERVOUS EXCITEMENT.
Brom. *140.* Calc. p. *167.*

IN PATIENTS SUBJECT TO PILES, DYSPEPSIA OR FLATULENCE.
Collin. *312.*

PANARITUM
chronic whitlow. Nat. sul. *585.*
Allium. 31.

PANCREAS
ACUTE INFLAMMATION.
Con. *328.*

BURNING IN.
Iris. *452.*

PARALYSIS
OF LEFT HALF OF FACE.
Alum. *32.*

OF LIMBS ON LEFT SIDE.
Alum. *35.*

OF INTESTINES.
Plumbum. Alum *35.*

OF ARMS AND HAND.
Caust. *229.*

OF EYES, MUSCLES, LIMBS.
Cocc. *294.*

OF THROAT.
Gels. Cocc. *294.*

OF DIAPHRAGM AND MUSCLES OF RESPIRATION.
Con. *331.*

OF TONGUE.
Cup. *345.*

OF LOWER EXTREMITIES.
Rhus radicans. Rhus *709.*

OF ALL MUSCLES.
Viscum. *868.*

PARTIAL PARALYSIS OF TONGUE OR LIMBS.
Arn. *88.*

VASO-MOTOR PARALYSIS.
Carbo v. *207,* Gels. *386.*

FACIAL PARALYSIS.
Caust. *222. 229.* Cocc. *294.*

HYPERAESTHESIA WITH LOSS OF POWER AS IN LANDRY'S DISEASES (ASCENDING PARALYSIS)
Plumbum (Cocc. *294*).

SPASTICITY WITH LOSS OF POWER.
Cocc. *295.*

FROM THE EXTREMITIES UPWARDS.
while the brain remains clear.
Con. 321.

AS RESULT OF ALUMINIUM
POISONING.
Alum. *40*.

CAUSED BY NERVOUS DISEASE.
Caust. *222*.

CAUSED BY EXPOSURE TO
COLD.
Caust. *222*.

ORIGINATING IN DISEASE OF
THE SPINAL CORD.
Cocc. *292*.

ORIGINATING IN LOCOMOTOR
ATAXIA.
Cocc. *292*.

AFTER DIPHTHERIA.
Cocc. *294*. Nat. mur *573*.

FROM NERVOUS EXHAUSTION,
SEXUAL EXCESSES, ANGER OR
EMOTION, PAIN.
Nat. mur. *573*.

AS RESULT OF OVER EXERTION.
Rhus. 710/1 715.

FROM COLD.
Sul. Caust. Rhus. *711*.

GRADUALLY APPEARING
PARALYSIS.
Caust. *229*.

WITHDRAWING OR TEARING
PAINS.
Cham. *242*.

PARALYTIC STIFFNESS OF
LIMBS.
Cocc. *291*. *294*. Graph. *400*.

PARALYTIC FEELING IN ARMS,
LEGS AND SPINE.
Aesc. *16*.

PARALYTIC WEAKNESS
(SLOWING DOWN OF ALL
ACTIVITIES OF BODY AND
MIND)
Cocc. *293*. Ver. alb. *857*.

SLOW TO RESPOND TO NERVOUS
IMPRESSIONS.
Cocc. *293*.

CANNOT EXPECTORATE —
SWALLOWS SPUTUM.
Con. *326*.

PARALYSIS AGITANS.
Mag. phos. *526*.

PARESIS.
Thuja. *823*.

PARAPLEGIA

SPASTIC.
Cocc. *295*. see SPINE.

PARESIS

slight or temporary paralysis.
see PARALYSIS.

PARONYCHIA

INFLAMMATION NEAR THE
NAIL. see FINGERS.

PAROTITIS

MUMPS. see MUMPS.

PECULIARITIES

SAYS SHE IS WELL, DESPITE
BEING ILL.
Arn. *85*. *88*.

DOES NOT FEEL AS SHE
GENERALLY DOES, BUT
CANNOT TELL WHY.
Brom *141*.

FEELS BED IS TOO HARD.
Arn. 86.

FEELS BETTER WHEN THINKING
OF HIS COMPLAINT.
Camph. *176.*

THOUGHT, SIGHT OR SMELL OF
FOOD TAKES AWAY HIS
APPETITE.
Ars. Sep. Cocc. Caust. *224.*
Colch. Cocc. *295.*

EVERY SYMPTOM < COFFEE.
Caust. *226.*

PRODUCES 'SPOONERISMS'
Caust. *226.*

WANTS TO EAT COAL.
Cicuta *265.*

WANTS TO EAT RAW POTATOES.
Cicuta *265.*

INCESSANT TALKING.
Cimic *272, 275. Lach. 498,*
Crot. *338.*

FEELING OF HOLLOWNESS IN
HEAD, CHEST OR ABDOMEN.
Cocc. *292.*

BAD EFFECTS FROM WINE OR
LIQUOR.
Coffea. *301.*

MUST LOOSEN CLOTHES.
Lyc. Ornithogalum. Nat. sul.
585 (Graph *398*)

MUST THROW OFF CLOTHES.
Hyos. *415.*

SHUDDERING.
Ipec. *444.*

PERIODICITY

ANNUALLY IN AUGUST.
coryza. Allium *30.*

ANNUALLY.
Tarent. *798.*

EVERY SPRING.
Crot. *337.*

EVERY TWO WEEKS.
Con. *322.* Iris. *449* even mental
symptoms. Con. *322.*

EVERY EIGHTH DAY.
Iris. *449.*

EVERY OTHER DAY.
China. *260.* Nat. mur. *574.*

REGULARLY.
Rhus. *711.*

SUNSET TO DAYLIGHT.
Syphilinum. (Med. *532*).

DAYLIGHT TO SUNSET.
Med. *532.*

< EVERY SPRING.
Lach. Rhus. Nat. sul. *580.*

< EVERY WINTER, SKIN
CRACKED, FINGERS
FISSURED.
Pet. 629. 630.

> IN SUMMER.
Pet. *629.*

HEADACHES EVERY 7TH DAY.
Sabad. Sil. Sul. Sang. *730* Sul.
784.

COUGH EVERY MORNING.
Alum. *36.*

DIARRHOEA ON RISING.
Nat. sul *580.*

DIARRHOEA AT 5 A.M.
Sul. *784.*

DIARRHOEA AT 9 A.M.
Nat. sul. *585.*

NEURALGIA EVERY 24 HOURS.
Sul. *784.*

WANTS PLENTY OF TIME TO DO
EVERYTHING.
Cocc. *294/5.*

< at night. Asaf. *105,* China
260. Merc. *537. 539.* Phyt. *651.*
Merc. *544* Ornithogalum.
(Graph. *398*) Ammon. carb.
43. Hepar. *406.*

< midnight. China *260,* Cocc.
296.

< after midnight. Ars. *96.*
Nat. mur. *574.*

< 1–2 a.m. (and 1–2 p.m.)
Ars. *96.*

< 2–3 a.m. colic. Nat. sul. *580.*

< 2–4 a.m. Kali bich. *461,*
Kali carb. *474.*

< 3 a.m. Ammon carb. *43, 46.*
Ant. tart. *66, 69. Bry. 146.*
Aeth. *18.*

< 3–5 a.m. Kali bich. *456.*

< 4–5 a.m. pneumonia or
asthma. *Nat. sul. 580. 585.*

< 7 a.m. neuralgia of
trigeminus. Nat. mur. *573.*

< 8–11 a.m. back muscles
stretched. Nat. mur. *573.*

< 9–10 a.m. chill. Nat. mur.
573.

< 10–11 a.m. Nat. mur. *569.*

< 9 a.m. Cham. *238.* Nat.
mur. *569.*

< 11 a.m. to 1 p.m. Hard
chill. Nat. mur. *573*

< on waking. Lach. (Gels.
384) Lyc. *519.*

< 4–8 p.m. *Lyc. 514.*

< 6–7 p.m. profuse urination.
Bry. *146.*

< 9 p.m. Bry. *146.*

< evenings. Allium *30, 32,*
Kali sul. *475.* Puls. *686.*

> 11 p.m. Borax. *134.*

PERIOSTITIS
INFLAMMATION OF BONE. see
BONES.

PERITONITIS
INFLAMMATION OF
PERITONEUM OR MEMBRANE
IN ABDOMINAL AND PELVIC
CAVITIES.
Bell. *117.* Tereb. *873.*

PETECHIA
SMALL SPOTS IN THE SKIN
RESEMBLING FLEA BITES. see
SKIN.

PEYER'S PATCHES
Dros *360.*

PHARYNX
Aesc. *15.*

MALIGNANT OR GANGRENOUS
PHARYNGITIS.
Caps. *203.*

STRINGY DISCHARGES IN
PHARYNGITIS.
Kali bich. *456.*

PARALYSIS OF . . .
Caust. *224*.

SPASMODIC CONSTRICTION OF.
Cham. *240*.

SEPTIC.
Kreos. *468*.

ITCHING IN . . .
Pet. *631*.

DRY, ROUGH. DARK RED.
Phyt. *651*.

HOT FEELING.
Phyt. *651*, Sang. *729*.

WITH REGURGITATION.
Phyt. *651*.

BURNING.
Sul. *782*.

PHOSPHATIC DIATHESIS
Calc. p. *167*.

PHTHISIS.
Caust. *224*. Chel. *248*. Agar.
21. Calc. p. *166*. Phos. *645*.
Sang. *728* Psor. *678*. Cimic.
271, Iod. *435*. Ipec. *446* Nat.
mur. *578* Nitric ac. *589*.
Theridion. *817*. Tub. *838*.
Thuja. *Bac.* Tub. *839*.

PHYMOSIS
CONTRACTION OF ORIFICE OF
PREPUCE SO THAT IT CANNOT
BE RETRACTED, A
CONGENITAL AFFECTION.
Arn. *89*.

PICROTOXIN
Cocc. *289*. *290/2*.

PILES (Haemorrhoids)
BURNING.
Kali carb. *469*, Lil. tig. *511*.
Mur. ac. *564*. Sul. *782*
(alternating with Nux. v.)
Med. *525*. Aesc. *12*. *14*. Caps.
201, *203*. Caust. *226*. Graph.
399.

< BY HEAT.
Ars. (Kali carb. *469*).

< BY SITTING IN COLD WATER.
Kali carb. *469*.

BLIND.
Nux. v. *605*. Sul. *789*. Med.
535. Aesc. *12*. Brom. *141*
Caps. *201*, Collin. *311/2*

BLIND OR BLEEDING.
Sul. *789*   Sul. alternating
with Nux. v. *606*.

BLEEDING.
Nit. ac. Aesc. *14*. Ammon.
carb. *43*, Caps. *201*. Collin.
311. *313* Ferr. phos. *380*. *Hyp.*
422. Tereb. *810*.

STAGNANT AND DRAGGING HER
DOWN.
Sepia *739*.

PAINFULLY SENSITIVE.
Sil. *753*.

SUPPRESSED.
Sul. *789*.

STITCHING, STINGING PAINS.
Bacillinum. (Tub. *834*).

SWOLLEN.
Caps. *201*. Mur. ac. *564*.

ITCHING AND THROBBING.
Caps. *201*, Mur. ac. *564*.

PROTRUDING.
Brom. *141*, Collin. *311/2*. Lil.
tig. *511*. Nitric ac. *592* Mur.
ac. *564*.

RAW.
Aloe, Aesc. *14*. Caust. *226*.

SORE.
Caust. *227*. Mur. ac. *563*.

DULL PAIN.
Collin *312*. Lyc. *518*.

ACHING.
Med. *535*. Aesc. *12*. Collin.
312.

PURPLISH.
Med. *535*. Aesc. *12*. *14*. Mur.
ac. *564*.

TENDENCY TO.
Caps. *200*. *205*.

AFTER RELIEF OF HEART
CONDITION.
Collin. *312*.

HAMMERING.
Lach. *497*.

PAINFUL TO TOUCH.
Mur. ac. *564*.

APPEAR SUDDENLY.
Mur. ac. *564*.

WITH:
constipation. Collin, *311/2*.
loss of appetite. Collin. *312*.
painful bleeding fissures.
Nitric ac. *588*. *592*.
ulcers. Paenonia. *624*.
black diarrhoeic stool. Brom.
141.
relaxation of veins. Calc. *157*.

bloody mucous stool. Caps.
201.
pain in the back. Caps. *201*.
pain in the abdomen. Caps.
201.
diarrhoeia. Collin. *311*.
alternate constipation and
diarrhoeia. Collin. *311*.

PROLAPSING AFTER EVERY
STOOL.
Nitric ac. *592*.

< FROM:
rheumatism. Abrot. *2*.
standing sitting, lying. Aesc.
14.
walking. Caust. *226*.
thinking of them. Caust *227*.
straining voice. Caust *226*.
after hard stool. Collin. *312*.
evenings and night. Collin.
312.
during pregnancy. Collin. *312*.

> FROM:
kneeling. Aesc. *14*.
carrying horse chestnuts in
pocket. Aesc. *12*.

PLEURISY
Bellis *127*. Bry. Borax. *132*.

WITH PRESSING SENSATION IN
BACK.
Abrot. *2*.

AFTER PLEURISY.
Acon. Bry. Ran. b. *699, 702*.

INFLAMMATORY.
Acon. *6*. Bry. *150*.

AFTER MECHANICAL INJURIES.
Arn. *90*.

PLEURITIC PAIN.
Borax. *136. Kali carb.* (Bry. *145*).

PLEURITIC PAIN < MOVEMENT.
Bry. *145*.

STITCHING PAIN IN PLEURA
< MOVEMENT.
Bry. *144*.

FIRST STAGE OF PLEURISY.
Ferr. phos. *380*.

< BETWEEN BREATHS.
Kali carb. *469*.

FROM SUDDEN EXPOSURE TO
COLD WHILE OVERHEATED.
Acon. Arn. Ran. b. *702*. Sul. *780* (after Acon).

AFTER STANDING ON COLD
GROUND.
Rhod. *704*.

PLEURODYNA
pain in the ribs. see CHEST.

PNEUMONIA
Phos. Nat. sul. Merc. (Bry. *146*).

WITH:
sleepiness – with dark red or purple face. Opium. Ant. tart. *63*.

with pale or cyanotic face. Atn. tart. *63*.

hepatization after. Ant. tart. *63*.

edges of eyelids covered with mucous. Ant. tart. *65*.

fetid expectoration. Carbo v. *211, 213*

fear of death. Acon. *6*.

diarrhoia and cramps. Cup. *346*.

expectoration of pure blood. Ferr. phos. *380*.

fan-like movement of alae nasi. Lyc. *520*.

frowning forehead. Lyc. *520*.

pressure in chest. *Phos. 646*.

great restlessness. Pyrogen *693*, Rhus *708, 712*.

fever at noon. Stram. *779*.

t.b. history. Tub. bov. 837.

red (or white) streak down centre of tongue. Ver. vir. *858*.

ref flushed face. Ver. vir. *858*.

high temperature. Ver vir. *858*.

sticking pains. Kali carb. (Bry. *145*) < movement. Bry. *145*.

ACUTE.
Ant. tart. *68*, Bell. *117*, Ferr. phos. *380*.

INCIPIENT.
Chel. *248. 251*.

LOW FORMS.
Ammon. carb. *45*.

PROSTRATION, WITH HEART
FAILURE AFTER . . .
Ferr. phos. *380*.

BRONCHO-PNEUMONIA OF
CHILDREN.
Ant. tart. *60/1. 68*. Bry. *146*.

PLEURO-PNEUMONIA, SOME
  PARALYSIS OF LUNGS.
  Ant. tart. *62, 68.*

RIGHT SIDED PAIN.
  Kali carb. (Bry. *145*).

'FLU' PNEUMONIA.
  Merc. *540.*

WITHOUT DEFINITE
  SYMPTOMS THAT WOULD
  CALL FOR ACON.
  Bry or Phos. Ferr. phos *381.*

TYPHOID PNEUMONIA.
  Sang. *730.*

< FROM:
  continual movement.
  Pyrogen. *693.*
  lying on inflamed side. Bel.
  (Bry. *145*).
  4 p.m. Lyc. *515.*
  right lung. Lyc. *520.*
  wet damp weather. Nat sul.
  581.

> FROM LYING ON INFLAMED
  SIDE.
  Bell. (Bry. *145*).

INFLAMMATION OF RIGHT
  LOWER LOBE.
  Kali carb. *470.*
  with offensive mouth and
  sweat. Merc. (Kali carb. *470*).
  with thirst for cold drinks.
  Phos. (Kali carb. *470*).

PNEUMOTHORAX
  Arn. 90.

POISONING
  by charcoal.
  Ammon carb. *44.*
  ptomaine. *Ars. 92.*

POLYCRESTS
AESCULUS.
  Aesc. *14.*

ARSENICUM.
  Ars. *95.*

BELLADONNA.
  Bell. *116.*

CALC. CARB.
  Calc. p. *169.*

CAUSTICUM.
  Caust. *221.*

IGNATIA.
  Ign. *424.*

LAC. CAN
  Lac. can. *488/9.*

LYCOPODEUM.
  Lyc. *520.*

NUX. VOM.
  Nux. *601.*

PHOSPHORUS.
  Phos. *640.*

PULSATILLA.
  Puls. *681.*

SANICULA.
  San. *732.*

SEPIA.
  Lac. can. *487.*

SILICA.
  Sil. *759.*

SULPHUR.
  Sul. *781*, Lac. Can. *487.*

PREGNANCY
(see also FEMALE SEX)

DISCOMFORT DURING . . .
Bellis *130*.

AFFECTIONS OF EARS
DURING . . .
Caps. *203*.

SHIVERS DURING FIRST
STAGE.
Cimic. *272/3*.

DIFFICULT WALKING.
Bellis. *131*.

SUFFERINGS DUE TO
MECHANICAL PRESSURE
SIMILAR TO BRUISING.
Arn. Bellis *131*.

FALSE LABOUR PAINS.
Calc. *162*, Vib. *863*.

VOMITING WITH NAUSEA
(MORNING SICKNESS).
Sepia *741*. Kreos *479*. Chel.
250. Ipec. *437*. Cimic. *271*.
Kali bich. *454*. Ferr. *370*. Iris.
452. San. *730*.

NERVOUSNESS.
Cimic. *274*.

TO PREVENT MISCARRIAGES.
Cimic. *276*. Vib. *863/4*.

RUSH OF BLOOD TO HEAD,
PALE FACE AND LOSS OF
CONSCIOUSNESS.
Glon. *389*.

FRIGHTFUL IMAGININGS IN
LATE PREGNANCY.
Kali br. *467*.

PRESSING AND BEARING
DOWN.
Sepia, Lil. tig. Kali carb. *473*.

WANTS BACK PRESSED.
Sepia, Kali carb. *473*.

LOCHIA OFFENSIVE,
EXCORIATING.
Kreos. *479*.

CONSTIPATION DURING . . .
Collin. *310. 312*.

THOUGHT OF FOOD TAKES
AWAY APPETITE.
Ars. Sep. Cocc. Caust. *224*.

CRAMP, IN TOES AND SOLES OF
FEET.
Calc. *162*.

CRAMP IN ABDOMEN AND
LEGS.
Vib. *862, 865*.

SIGHT OF WATER MAKES ONE
VOMIT.
Phos. *644*.

SWELLING AND STIFFNESS OF
HANDS AND FEET.
San. *735*.

SENSATION THAT OS UTERI IS
OPENING.
Lach. San. *735*.

TOOTHACHE OF PREGNANCY.
Sepia. *741*.

CHLOASMA.
Sepia. *741*.

DURING LABOUR:
becomes blind. Cup *344*.
suffocating spells and
convulsions. Hyoc. *414*.

TO FACILITATE LABOUR.
Borax. *132*.

PRIAPISM
PERSISTENT ERECTION OF
PENIS, LEWDNESS,
LICENTIOUSNESS.
Canth. *193, 198* Picric ac. *657.*

PROSOPALGIA
FACIAL NEURALGIA.
Caust. *227.*

PRURITIS
ITCHING. see SKIN.

PTOSIS
DROOPING OF EYELIDS
PARTICULARLY. see EYES.
Sepia *739.*

PUDENDA
EXTERNAL GENITALS.
Carbo v. *212.* Graph. *399.*
Kreos. *479.*

PURPURA
PURPLE SPOTS. see SKIN.

PUS
WITH A VENT.
Calc. s. 171.
YELLOW AND THICK.
Calc. s. *171/2.*
IN URINE.
Calc. s. *172.*

PYAEMIA
BLOOD POISONING FORMING
ABSCESSES.
Phos. *645.*

PYELITIS
INFLAMMATION OF PELVIS OF
KIDNEY. see KIDNEYS

PYOTHORAX
PUS IN THORAX. see CHEST.

PYREXIA
FEVER.
Ipec. *433.* see FEVERS.

PYROSIS
WATERBRASH.
Alum. *37.*

Q

QUININE
Calc. *163.* Ign. *426.* Ipec. *440.*
Nat. mur. *569.*

R

RAILWAY SPINE
CONCUSSION OF THE SPINAL
CORD.
Bellis. *130.*

RASH
MILITARY.
Ail. *26.* Puls. Ail. *29.*
pemphigus. Ail. *27.*
red spots. Ail. *28. see ALSO
SKIN.*

RECTUM AND ANUS

SORE.
Aesc. *12.*

BURNING.
Collin. *311/2.* Aesc. *12. 14.*
Canth. *193. 195.* Caps. *199, 201*
Carbo v. *212.*

ITCHING.
Graph. *399.* Aesc. *12.* Carbo v.
212. Cina. *280.* Collin. *311.*
Nitric ac. *591.* Sul. *789.*

FEELS FULL OF SMALL STICKS.
Aesc. *12.* Collin. Aesc. *14. 15.*
Collin. 311/2.

FEELING OF SPLINTERS.
Nitric ac. Aesc. *14.* Iris. *450*
Nitric ac. *593.*

DRY.
Aesc. *14.*

CONSTRICTED.
Aesc. *14.* Borax. *134.*

INACTIVE.
Alum. *36.*

FEELS PARALYSED.
Alum. *36.* Collin. *312.*

POWERLESS.
Anac. *48.*

INFLAMED.
Borax. *132.* Kali carb. *473.*

BURING AND APHTHAE
Borox. *132.*

POLYPS.
Calc. p. *167.*

TENESMUS.
Caps. *201.* Colch. *307.*

PAIN AFTER STOOL.
Colch. *309.* Graph. *399.* Ign.
431. Merc. *543.* Nux. v. *605.*

TEARING WHEN NOT URINATING.
Ruta. *721.*

TEARING, STITCHING WHEN SITTING.
Ruta. *721.*

FEELS CONSTRICTED.
Cactus. (Gels. *384*).

PRESSURE IN RECTUM AND ANUS.
Lil, tig. *509.*

PAIN WITH STOOL AS IF RECTUM WOULD BE TORN ASUNDER.
Nitric ac. *591.* Plumbum. *664.*

ULCER ON PERINEUM BY ANUS.
Paeonia. *622, 624.*

FEELS AS IF FULL.
Anac. *48.* Aesc. *122, 124.*

PAIN WITH STOOL AS IF RECTUM WOULD BE TORN ASUNDER.
Nitric ac. *591.*

PAIN IN RECTUM AND ANUS AFTER EATING.
Nux. v. *605.*

PAIN IN RECTUM AND ANUS AFTER EXERTING MIND.
Nux. v. *605.*

RECTUM:
heat in . . . Paeonia. *622.*
itching. Sul. *789.*
crawling in . . . Tereb. *812.*
prolapse of . . . Ruta *719. 721.*
Sepia *748.*
burning. Tereb. *810. 812.*

as of boiling lead passing through. Thuja *829*.

ANUS:

pressure in . . . Collin. *311*.

coldness in . . . Con. *330*.

remains open. Gels. *382*.

prolapse of . . . Collin. *310*. *313*,

Ferr. *373*, Ruta. *719*.

burning in . . . after stool. Iris. *450*, Paeonia. *624*.

painfully closed. Lyc. *518*.

constriction round prolapsed . . . Mez. *554*.

itching of . . . Nat. phos. *576*, Nitric ac. *591*. Paeonia. *622*.

raw. Nat. phos. *576*.

offensive moisture round. Nitric ac. *588* Sil. *753*. Paeonia. *624*.

purple. Paeonia *624*.

swelling and itching. Paeonia. *624*.

burning. Phos. *643*. *Sil. 753*. Paeonia *624*. Tereb. *810* Sul. *782*. *789*.

itching while sitting. Staph. *763*.

reddens, with itching. Sul. *782*.

excoriation about . . . Sul. *789*.

bleeding from . . . Sul. *789*.

fissured. Thuja. *819*. *828*.

with warts and condylomata. Thuja. *828/9*.

constricted. Plumbum. *664*. *670*.

sense of heavy weight in . . . Sepia *748*.

feeling of hammers in . . . Lach. *498*.

HAEMORRHAGES FROM . . < AUTUMNAL COLD DAMP WEATHER.
Colch. *309*.

FISSURES IN . . .
Calc. p. *168*, Caust. *224*. Cham. *240*, Sil. *753*. Paeonia *622*. *624*.

SENSATION OF LUMP OR PLUG IN.
Anac. *51*. Kali br. *461*. Sepia. *741*.

FISTULO IN ANO.
Calc. p. *166*. *168*. Kali carb. *473*. Sil. *753*. *759*. Lach. *497*.

FEELS FULL BUT WITHOUT ACTUAL CONSTIPATION.
Aesc. *15*.

SENSATION OF ITS BURSTING.
Agar. *22*.

STRAINING AFTER STOOL.
Merc. cor Agar. *22*.

REQUIRES STRAINING.
Alum. *36*.

SENSATION OF EXCORIATION.
Alum. *36*. LYc. *518*.

SENSATION OF CRAWLING IN . . . AS IF FROM WORMS.
Alum. *37*.

BLOOD AFTER EVACUATION.
Alum. *37*.

PROTRUSION DURING STOOL.
Ant. crud. *55*. Ign. *430*.

163

THICKENING OF MUCOUS
MEMBRANES.
Borax. *134.*

FISTULA ALTERNATING WITH
CHEST SYMPTOMS.
Calc. p. *166/8.*

NAUSEA FELT IN.
Ruta. (Cocc. *299*).

PAIN IN RECTUM AND ANUS.
Colch. *309.* Ign. *429, 431.* Mez.
553.

RESPIRATION.
see CHEST.

RETINITIS
INFLAMMATION OF THE
RETINA. see EYES.

RHAGADES
CHAPS OR FISSURES OF THE
SKIN.
Sul. *790.*

RHEUMATISM
Nat. phos. (Cina *278*)

PAINFUL.
Sal. ac. *725.* Abrot. *2.* Ledum.
504.

INFLAMMATORY.
Merc. *539,* Abrot. *2.* Ant.
crud. *52.* Aur. *109.*

ACUTE.
Aur. *109,* Bell. *125.* Ledum.
504. Tub. *837.* Colch. *304. 308*
Ferr. phos. *380.* Ver. vir. *860.*

CHRONIC.
Bell. *125.* Ledum. *504.* Pet.
630, Rhod. *704.*

CHRONIC FROM LATENT
GONORRHEA.
Med. *533.*

WITH CHRONIC CATARRH.
Cistus *288.*

ARTICULAR (OF JOINTS).
Ferr. phos. *380.* Rhus. *709.*
Sal. ac. *724.*

RHEUMATOID ARTHRITIS
BEGINNING AT THE
MENOPAUSE.
Caul. *220.* Cimic. *274.*

INTERCOSTAL.
Ran. b. 701.

SWOLLEN, HOT, PALE.
Ledum *504.* Sal. ac. *725.*

WITH DIAGONAL PAINS.
Agar. *22.*

RHEUMATIC FEVER.
Bell. *125.* Ign. *429.*
never well since, or result
of . . . Streptococcin. (Morb.
561).

SHIFTING PAINS.
Colch. *309,* Puls. Kali sul. *475.*

WANDERING PAINS.
Lac. can. Rhod. *704.*

WANDERING FROM JOINT TO
JOINT.
Rhod. *704.* Colch. *304.* Puls.
686.

STIFFNESS ON RISING.
Nat. phos. *577.*

MOVING FROM LOWER LIMBS
UPWARDS.
Ledum. *506*.

METASTASIS FROM JOINTS TO
HEART.
Nat. mur. *575*

ALTERNATING WITH:
haemoptysis. Ledum. *502*.
catarrh. Kali bich. *454*.
gastric symptoms. Kali bich.
461.
dysentery. Kali br. Abrot. *3*.

WITH EXTREME TENDERNESS
OF SOLES OF FEET.
Ant. crud. *57*.

IN PLACES LEAST COVERED
WITH FLESH.
Sang. *730*.

BEFORE SWELLING
COMMENCES.
Abrot. *2*.

> CARRYING HORSE
CHESTNUT.
Aesc. *16*.

IN NECK, ONLY ON MOVEMENT.
Acon. *9, 10*.

RHEUMATIC STIFF NECK.
Bell. 125.

< GETTING HEAD WET.
Bell. *125*.

< EXPOSED TO DRAUGHT.
Bell. *125*.

IN JOINTS.
Calc. p. *166*.

IN JOINTS.
Calc. p. *166*.

IN SMALL JOINTS AND MUSCLES.
Caul. *217. 219*.

OF PHALANGEAL AND
METACARPAL JOINTS.
Caul. *215*.

OF SPINE.
Caul. *219*.

OF MUSCLES AND NERVES.
Cimic. *274*.

IN SHOULDER.
Sul. *780*.

IN RIGHT SHOULDER.
Sang. *730*.

IN RIGHT DELTOID.
Urtica *846*.

WITH:
red blush over joints. Colch.
304.
hyperaesthesia. Colch. *304*.
numbness. Kreos. *482*.

IN CHILDREN.
Nat. phos. *575*.

MUSCULAR.
Rhus. *709*.

DEFORMITIES AND
CONTRACTIONS.
Caust. 230.

VIOLENT PAINS DRIVE OUT OF
BED.
Cham. *241*.

COME AND GO.
Colch. *309*.

< AT REST AND SITTING.
Agar. *22*.

> MOVING.
Agar. *22*.

< COLD WEATHER.
Calc. p. *166, Caust. 223.*

> IN SPRING.
Calc. p. *166.*

> WARM WET WEATHER.
Caust. 223.

< WET WEATHER.
Rhod. *704.*

< COLD DAMP WEATHER.
Colch. *304, 308.* Phyt. *651.*

< DRY WEATHER.
Caust *233.*

< SLIGHTEST MOTION.
Ferr. phos. *380.*

< AT NIGHT.
Ledum. *504.* Sang. *729.*

< WARMTH OF BED.
Ledum. *504.* Merc. *539.*

< TOUCH OF ANYTHING COLD.
Sal. ac. *725.*

< DURING REPOSE.
Rhus. *709.*

RESTLESSNESS
Ars. 92. Coffea 300. *Pyrogen 694.* Kreos *481.*

EXCESSIVE.
Acon. *8*, Ail. *26*, Arn. *86*, Dros. *361.*

AT NIGHT.
Acon. *8.*

ANXIOUS RESTLESSNESS.
Acon. Ars. Arn. *86*, Ign. *432.*

WITH PROSTRATION, OUT OF ALL PROPORTION TO APPARENT CONDITION.
Ars. *92.*

DUE TO CHOREA.
Cimic. *276.*

DUE TO WORMS.
Cina. *281.*

CRIES OUT IN SLEEP.
Apis. Cina *281.*

HOT BLOODED.
Iod. *436.*

COLD BLOODED.
Ars. (Iod. *436*).

FEELS MOVEMENT WOULD HELP.
Rhus, Arn. *86.* Ferr. *371.*

DESIRES TO GO FROM PLACE TO PLACE.
Tub. San. *733* Calc. p. *166.*

NOTE – ARSENICUM MAY BE THE RIGHT REMEDY EVEN WITHOUT RESTLESSNESS. see SEPIA 745.

RICKETS
Calc *154/6 159/60* Calc. p. *165 167* (rachitis) *170* Ferr. phos *375* Silica *757* Theridion. *817.*

S

SACRUM
BRUISED PAIN.
Acon. *10.*

HEAVINESS AND LAMENESS IN SACRO-ILEAC REGION.
Aesc. *12.*

PAIN < SITTING.
Agar. *22.* Aesc. *12.*

< RISING FROM SITTING.
Aesc. *12.*

< STOOPING.
Aesc. *12.* Kali bich. *460.*

< WALKING.
Aesc. *12.*

SEVERE ACHE.
Agar. *22. 24.*

AS IF SOMETHING CRACKED
WHEN STOOPING.
Kali bich. *460.*

PAIN IN SMALL SPOT, < NIGHT.
Kali bich. *460.*

PAIN IN COCCYX.
Kali bich. *458. 460.*

< RIDING IN CARRIAGE.
Nux. mosc. *597.*

SANTONIN
Cina *278, 284.*

SARCOCELE
Aur. *107.*

SATYRIASIS
MORBID OVERPOWERING
SEXUAL DESIRE IN MEN —
CORRESPONDING TO
NYMPHOMANIA IN WOMEN.
Cann. *183.* Canth. *196, 198.*
Picric ac. *657.* see
GENITALIA.

SCARS
OLD SCARS TURNING PURPLE.
Asaf. *104.*

THREATEN TO SUPPURATE.
Asaf. *104.*

BECOME VEINOUS, PAINFUL
AND TURNING BLACK.
Asaf. *104.*

SCAR TISSUE. GRAPH.
Sil. Dros. *357.*

SCARS OF GLANDS.
Dros. *359.*

BREAKING DOWN SCAR TISSUE.
Sil. *752.*

'ULCERS OUT' FOREIGN BODIES.
Sil. *752.*

SCIATICA
see LEGS.

SCINDE'S boils
OF MALARIAL ORIGIN?
Urtica *847.*

SCIRRHUS
HARD TUMOUR. see CANCER.

SCORBICULOUS CORDI
Ornithogalum. *619.* Puls. *684.*

SCROFULA
CONSTITUTIONAL WEAKNESS,
ALSO KNOWN AS THE
TUBERCULAR CONSTITUTION.
Calc. *163.*

SCYBALA
VERY HARD STOOLS IN
AGGRAVATED
CONSTIPATION.
Plumbum *666.*

SEASICKNESS
see VOMITING

SENSATIONS

TINGLING.
Acon. *8*. Ail. *27*.

HAMMERING.
Lach. Acon. *8*.

STITCHING LIKE HOT
NEEDLES.
Ars. Acon. *8*.

STITCHING AND STABBING.
Acon. *8*.

on movement. Bry. Spig.
Acon. *8*.

independent of movement.
Kali carb. Acon. *8*.

OF STITCHES ON TONGUE.
Acon. *9*.

SHIVERING > MOVING.
Dros. *362*.

< moving. Nux. (Dros. *362*).

< when at rest. Dros. 362.

NUMBNESS.
Acon. *11*.

FORMICATIONS.
Acon. *11*.

OF FALLING.
Bell. *124*. Vib. *865*.

OF RED HOT IRON AT VERTEX.
Crot. casc. (Crot. *339*).

OF SUFFOCATION.
Vib. *886*.

OF BEING TRANSPARENT.
Cann. *185*.

OF GRADUALLY SWELLING.
Cann. *185*. *187*.

OF WATER IN THE CHEST.
Crot. casc. (Crot *339*).

OF FACE GROWING LARGER.
Acon. *9*.

OF A DUAL EXISTENCE.
Cann. *184/89*.

OF SHORTENING RIGHT LIMB.
Crot. casc. (Crot. *339*).

OF ARMS AND LEGS CROWDING
HIM.
Pyrogen. *691*. *693*.

OF COLD WATER ON BODY.
Ran. b. *701*.

OF UPPER PART OF BODY
floATING IN AIR.
Viscum. *868*.

OF OPENING IN STOMACH,
THROUGH WHICH AIR
PASSES.
Crot. casc. (Crot. *339*).

OF PEG STICKING IN MIDDLE OF
LIVER.
Crot. casc. (Crot. *339*).

OF A POLICEMAN COMING IN.
Kali brom. Hyos. *411*.

OF SOMETHING SITTING BY HIS
SIDE.
Hyos. *412*. Pyrogen. *691*.

OF SOMEONE FOLLOWING.
Lach. Med. Staph. *766*.

OF BUGS RUNNING OVER LIPS.
Graph. *399*, Borax. *136*.

OF INSECTS CRAWLING OVER
SURFACE.
Ledum. *507*, Mez. *554*.

OF ANTS RUNNING OVER CHEST.
Mez. *554*, Phos. ac. *638*.

OF ANTS RUNNING THROUGH
THE WHOLE BODY.
Cistus. *287.*
< lying down. Cistus. *287.*
> fresh air. Cistus. *287.*

OF SOMETHING ALIVE IN THE
BODY.
Crocus. Thuja. (Cocc. *295*)
Cycl. *351* Tarent. *801*, Crocus.
Thuja. Theridion. Pall. *625*
Pet. *632*. Sang. *730* Thuja. *816.*
820.

OF SOMEONE ELSE IN BED.
Pet. *632/3.*

OF 'COVERING' THE WHOLE
BED.
Pyrogen. *691. 696.*

OF BED BEING TOO SMALL.
Sul. *784.*

BED FEELS TOO HARD.
Arn. *90*, Pyrogen *695.* Bapt.
115. Dros. *362.*

AS IF THE BED WERE TIPPING
OVER.
Ars. *100.*

AS IF ONE WERE FALLING OUT
OF BED.
Crot. casc. (Crot. *339*).

AS IF HEART STOPPED.
Cicuta *263/4 269.*

AS IF BRAIN MOVED IN THE
SKULL.
Ars. *100.*

AS IF A HOOP OR BAND WERE
ROUND A PART.
Anac. *48.*

AS IF HE WERE IN A STRANGE
PLACE.
Opium. Cicuta. *264.*

AS IF TIME AND SPACE
EXTENDED.
Cann. *184* Bapt. *113.*

AS IF THE ROOM WERE TOO
SMALL.
Cycl. *351.*

AS IF TONGUE WERE SCALDED.
Plat. *662.*

AS IF LEGS WERE MADE OF
WOOD.
Thuja. *820.*

AS IF BODY WERE BRITTLE.
Thuja. *820.*

AS IF COLD WATER RAN DOWN
OUTSIDE OESOPHAGUS.
Ver. alb. *857.*

AS IF DAMP CLOTHING WAS ON
ARMS AND LEGS.
Sepia. Ver. vir. *862.*

AS IF BAG OF WATER TURNS
WHEN TURNING OVER IN
BED.
Ornithogalum (Graph. *398*).

AS IF A BLACK CLOUD
ENVELOPED HER.
Cimic. *272.*

AS IF DRUNK.
Mez. *554.*

AS IF SKULL WOULD SPLIT.
Mez. *554*

AS IF HOT WATER POURED
FROM BREAST INTO
ABDOMEN.
Sang. *730.*

AS IF WORM WERE CRAWLING
IN STOMACH.
Cocc. *295*.

AS IF SOMETHING WERE ALIVE
IN THE HEAD.
Crot. casc. (Crot. *339*).

AS IF DOGS GNAWED FLESH
AND BONES.
Nitric ac. *593*. Stram. *776*,
Pall. *627*

AS IF CRAWLING FROM FLEAS.
Pall. *625*.

AS IF SPIDERS CRAWLED OVER
HAND.
Viscum. *868*.

IMAGINES — HE SEES RATS,
DOGS AND CATS RUNNING
ACROSS THE ROOM.
Aeth. *19*.

bugs crawling over bed. Ars.
100.

mouse running up leg and
arms. Calc. *155*. Cimic. *272*.
Sul. *784*.

she sees strange objects.
Cimic. *273*.

she sees ghosts during day.
Ars. *100*.

house is full of thieves. Ars.
100.

she has lost the affection of
friends. Aur. *106*.

he is not fit for this world.
Aur. *106*.

she is 'scattered about'. Bapt.
115

things and people are black.
Stram. *778*.

HORRIFYING IMAGINING.
Stram. *775–777*.

EVERYTHING EXAGGERATED.
Cann. *178*.

WITH INTENSE EXALTATION.
Cann. *178*.

MULTIPLE DELUSIONS.
Pyrogen. *691*.

OBJECTS SEEM VERY LARGE.
Hyos. *413*.

OBJECTS SEEM VERY SMALL.
Plat. (Hyos. *413*).

SEES EVERYTHING IN
APPARENT MOTION WITH
SOLID OBJECTS SHINING
THROUGH.
Cycl. *349*.

WAVING SENSATION IN THE
BRAIN.
Cimic. *272*.

SEES DEATH AS GIGANTIC
BLACK SKELETON.
Crot. *339*.

HEARS STRANGE VOICES.
Crot casc. (Crot *339*).

FANCIES HER EYES ARE
FALLING OUT.
Crot. casc. (Crot. *339*).

SENSATION IN ABDOMEN AT
NIGHT CAUSING ENDLESS
STRETCHING.
Plumbum. *670*.

FEELING OF RAT RUNNING UP
LEG.
Ail. *29*.

FEELING OF FACE COVERED
WITH COBWEBS.
Alum. *39*. Graph. *395, 399*.

Borax. *136.*

FEELS LIKE A CHILD.
Cicuta. *264.*

FEELS SHE IS SWAYING.
Cicuta. *264.*

ITCHING BURNING FEELING AS A RESULT OF SLIGHT MENTAL EMOTION.
Bry. *147.*

FEELS AS IF FALLING FROM A HEIGHT.
Thuja. Bell. *122.* Caps. *204.*

SENSITIVITY
see also MOTION and MODALITIES.

HYPERAESTHESIA – OVER SENSITIVENESS.
Caps. *205.* China *258,* Cocc. *294* Plumbum. (Cocc. *294*) Colch. *309.* Hepar. *402.* Nux. v. *602.* Ars. *96,* Hepar. Asaf. *104.* Bell. *123.* Borax. *134.* Dros. *353* Hepar (Calc. s. *172*) Cann. *190.* Cann. China *260.* Cup. *346.* Acon. Cham. Nux. v. Ign. *425.*

HYPERAESTHESIA WITH LOSS OF POWER.
Cocc. *294.* Plumbum. *663, 669.*

of the skin. (desires to be naked) Hyos. *412. 415.*

complete insensibility, deep coma. Opium. *616.*

EXCESSIVE UNEASINESS. NUX. v. *602.*

TO SMELL.
Bell. *122/3* Colch. *306/7* Mur. ac. *564.* Nux. v. *602.*

TO TASTE.
Bell. *123.* Mur. ac. *564.*

TO HEARING.
Bell. *123.* Mur. ac. *564.*

TO LIGHT.
Bell. *123.* Mur. ac. *564.* Nat. sul. *581.*

TO TOUCH.
Hepar. Calc. s. *172,* China *258,* Coffea. *301,* Hepar. *402.*

TO DRAUGHTS.
Hepar. Calc. s. *172.* Hepar. *402.*

TO CLOTHES.
Sul. Calc. s. *172.*

TO PAIN.
Cocc. *294.* Hepar *402.* Cham. Lyc. *516.* Nux. *604.*

TO OPEN AIR.
Sul. *791.*

TO COLD.
Dulc. *365.* Hepar. *402.*

TO COLD AIR.
Hepar. *402. 406/7.*

TO NOISE.
Ptelea. *680.* Acon. *9.* Opium. *613.* Sepia. *741.* Nux. v. *602* Lach. *495.* Coffea. (Colch. *306*). Sil. *752.* Nat sul. *581* Theridion. (Picric. ac. *655*) *815, 817,* Sil. *753.*

TO TOUCH.
Theridion. (Picric ac. *655*) *Ran. b. 701,* San. *736.*

TO SMELL OF COOKING.
Ars. Cocc. Colch. Dig. Ipec. Thuja. Sepia *741.*

TO SMELL, SIGHT OR THOUGHT
OF FOOD.
Colch. *306/8*.

TO COLOUR.
Tarent. *798*.

TO HARMLESS WORDS WHICH
OFFEND.
Staph. *767*.

TO SCRATCHING OF LINEN OR
SILK.
Ferr. Tarax. Asarum.
(Theridion. *818*).

TO MOVEMENT.
Nux. v. *602*. (see MOTION).

TO SURROUNDINGS.
Lach. *495*. (cf. Opium.
Lyssin).

TO MUSIC.
Sepia. *741*, Sul. *784*.

MUSIC MAKES HER WEEP.
Graph. *398*.

MUSIC MAKES HER WILD.
Nast. sul. *581*.

WOMEN WHO BLUSH EASILY.
Ferr. *372*.

TO INHALED COLD AIR.
Aesc. *15*. China *260*, Cistus
288.

WHOLE BODY, TO TOUCH.
Acon. *11*.

VERY FASTIDIOUS.
Nux. Ars. *96*.

EXCESSIVELY SORE.
Arn. Bapt. Pyrogen. *690*.

THROWS OFF COVERS WHEN
COLD.
Camph. *175* Calc. s. *172*,
Secale (Camph. *175*)

CANNOT ENDURE
UNCOVERING.
Hepar (CaLc. s. *172*).

CANNOT ENDURE
UNCOVERING WHEN HOT.
Camph. *175*.

SEPSIS

MOST RAPID.
Lach. Tarent. Anthracinum.
Pyrogen. Sepsin. Crot. *334*.

LESS RAPID.
Hepar. Sil. Merc. Crot. *334*.

SEXUAL

DESIRE INCREASED.
Calc. *161*, Canth. *198*.

WEAK AFTER INDULGENCE.
Calc. *161*.

EJACULATION TARDY.
Calc. *161*.

IMPOTENCE.
Calc. *161*, Med. *534*.

CONSEQUENCES OF ONANISM.
Calc. *161*, Ferr. *371*, Phos ac.
638. Tarent *802* Carb. v. *212*.

TOO FREQUENT COITUS.
Calc. *161*.

NOCTURNAL INVOLUNTARY
EMISSIONS.
Calc. *161*.

HEADACHES WHEN DEPRIVED
OF SEXUAL INTERCOURSE.
Camph. *176*.

AFTER SEXUAL EXCESS.
Carbo v. *212*.

BAD EFFECTS FROM
SUPPRESSED DESIRE, OR
EXCESSIVE INDULGENCE.
Con. *327.*

HYSTERIA AND
HYPOCHONDRIASIS FROM
ABSTINENCE FROM SEXUAL
INTERCOURSE.
Con. *328.*

SHINGLES
see HERPES

SHOCK
TO PREVENT AFTER EFFECTS.
Arn. 87.

FOR EFFECTS OF.
Camph. *176.*

SIDES
LEFT-SIDED.
Asaf. *103,* Lach. (Crot. *335)*
493, Arg. nit, Caps. Cina.
Clematis. Crocus.
Euphorbium. Graph. Kreos,
Lach. Oleander Phos.
Selenium. Sep. Stan. Asaf.
104. Caps. *204.*

LEFT-SIDED PAINS:
high up under clavicle. Myrtis
Communis (Cean. *232*).
a little lower. Sumbul.
lower still. Acidum fluoricum.
further left. Acidum
Oxalicum.
further right. Aurum
under left breast. Cimic.
deep behind ribs. China.

Chel. Berb. Chin. sul.
Conium. Cean. americanus.

RIGHT-SIDED.
Ammon carb. Ars. Aur. Bapt.
Bell. Bovista, Canth. Lyc.
Puls. Ran. b. Sars. Sec. Sul.
ac. Asaf. *104.* Chel. *248* Crot.
335, Mag. phos. *525.*

FROM SIDE TO SIDE AND BACK
AGAIN.
Lac. can. Ant. crud. *52.*

FROM LEFT TO RIGHT.
Lach. Ant. crud. *52,* Allium
30.

FROM RIGHT TO LEFT.
Lyc. Ant. crud. *52.* Chel. *248.*

ONE SIDE OR THE OTHER.
Apis, Arg. nit. Bry. Calc.
Chel, Coloc, Ran. s. Sul. Asaf.
104, Kali bich. *455.*

SIGHING
INVOLUNTARY.
Calc. p. *167.*

SINCIPUT
FOREPART OF THE HEAD OR
SKULL.
Cina 282, see HEADACHES.

SKIN
SCARLET FEVER, SCARLATINA.
Arum. tryph. *29,* (Ail. *29*).

DERMATITIS.
Bellis. *130.*

BARBER'S ITCH.
Nat. sul. 582.

BROWN SPOTS.
Chloasma. Sepia. *743.*

BROWN SPOTS WITH
LEUCORRHEA.
Sepia. *743.*

CARBUNCLES.
Tarent. *805,* Kreos. *482.*

CHAPS.
Pet. *630.*

COMEDONES – BLACKHEADS.
Sul. *792.*

CRUSTA LACTEA OF BABIES.
Dulc. *364/5,* Mez. *555.* Mez.
Graph *396.* Calc. *160.*

EPITHELIOMA.
Kali sul. *476.* Kreos. *482.*
Sepia *747* Merc. *540.*

ERYTHEMA, BURNING
SMARTING, ITCHING.
Ran. b. *701.*
exanthemata. Pet. *629,* Rhus.
715. Ars. *97.*

ICHTHYOSIS, WITH EVIL
ODOUR.
Psor. *675.*

IMPETIGO.
Meg. *555.*

INTERTRIGO.
Sepia. 744.

LUPUS.
Phyt. *649.*

PEMPHIGUS.
Ran. b. *700, 702.*

PITYRIASIS.
Phyt. *649.*

PRURITIS.
Canth. *196.* Tarent. *802.*

PSORIASIS.
Puls *682.* Graph. *398,* Iris. *449.*
Kali sul. *477,* Phos. *649.*
of palms. Pet. *632,* Kali sul.
477. Phos. *649.*

TINEA CAPITIS.
Caust. 226, Iris. *449, 451,*
Phys. *649.*

TINEA KERION.
Mez. *547.*

PURPURA.
Phos. ac. *639.* Phos. *645* Tereb.
812.

SKIN WITHERS.
Plumbum. *665.*

YELLOWISH.
Plumbum. *666. 669*

EVERY SCRATCH FESTERS AND
ULCERATES.
Sil. *751.*

WILL NOT HEAL.
Sil. *751.*

ITCHINGS – EVERYWHERE.
Sul. *792.*
< at night, morning after
waking. Sul. *792.*
< in bed. Sul. *792.*
on head. Ant. crud. *52* Rhus.
Anac *50,* Canth. *196,* Chel.
251, Ipec. *438.*
with pricking on scalp. Cycl.
350.
leading to ulcers. Kali bich.
461.
violent. Kreos. *480.* Mez *554/6*
when body gets warm. Psor.
678. 673.

on bends of elbows. Sepia.
743.

with dry rough scaly skin.
Hepar. Sil. Sul. *782*.

< finger joints, followed by
boils. Psor. *676*.

BURNINGS – OF SKIN OF WHOLE
BODY.
Sul. *792*.

any boils, abscesses, felons,
swellings which are bluish
(Anthracinum Sil. Lach.)
with intense burning pains.
Terent. *805/6*.

inflammations. Arn. *90*,
Canth. *195*.

red, itchy, burning. Agar. *23*,
Stram, *775*, Bell. *117, 119, 123*.
Canth. *196*. Caps. *202*.

PURPLISH.
Mur. ac. *565*, Terent. *798*.

DIRTY UNHEALTHY.
Nat. mur. *571*, Psor. *676*.

UNHEALTHY.
Borax. *133*, Hepar. Calc. s.
172. Hepar. *401*.

ULCERATES EASILY.
Borax. *133*, Hepar. (Calc. s.
172) Hepar *401*. Ant. crud. *58*.

EVERY LITTLE INJURY
SUPPURATES.
Sil. Hepar *401*. Sil. Graph.
Merc. Pet. Hepar *403, 406*. Sil.
754.

FORMICATION.
Sul, *792*.

NETTLERASH.
Sul. *792*. Dulc. *363/4*. Nat.
mur. *573*.

URTICARIA, INTENSE, WITH
BURNING, ITCHING,
NUMBNESS, SWELLING,
OEDEMA, VESICATION.
Urtica *845*, Apis. *73*. Rhus.
715.

ERYTHEMA NODOSUM.
Kali br. *466*.

ERYSIPELAS, AMBULATING,
CHANGING FROM SIDE TO
SIDE AND BACK AGAIN.
Lac. can. *490*.

ERUPTIONS:
only on covereed parts.
Thuja. *829*.

(note – sweat on UNcovered
parts)

as result of vaccinations.
Thuja. *826*.

alternating with other
ailments e.g. asthma. Ars.
Sul. *782*.

burning. Sul. *782*.

suppressed, resulting in
scrofulous chronic diseases.
Sul. *791*.

pustular. Tarent. *802*.

vesicular. Rhus. *716*.

bleed easily. Psor. *678*.

tettery, humid, Sepia. *743*.

itch violently Pet. *631*.

thin and watery. Pet. *631*.

gluey, sticky, viscid. Graph.
(Pet. *631*).

oozing. Graph. *395*.

in bends of elbows, groin etc. Sepia. Graph. *396*.

> when tendency to obesity. Graph. *397*.

dry, itching. Sul. (Hepar. *403*).

moist suppurating, sensitive to touch. Hepar. *403, 406*.

suppurate, Hepar. Pet. *630*. Phys. *649*.

suppressed. Ipec. *438*.

only on covered parts. Ledum. *507*.

only on UNcovered parts. Thuja. (Ledum. *507*).

on scalp. Mez. *551*.

on face. Mez. *552*.

offensive, sickening odour Psor. *673*.

itching and burning. Alum. *39*.

< warmth of bed. Alum. *39*.

rough, dry. Alum. *39*.

similar to blisters. Caust. *230*, Rhus. *715*.

starting up 4 p.m. Lyc *515*.

spreading over whole body. Ledum. *502*. Rhus. *715*.

penetrating mouth, causing coughing Ledum. *502*.

WARTS.
Thuja. *819*.

large, pedunculated. Caust. *230*.

suppressed. *Thuja. 820*.

< bathing. Psor. *673*.

< WARMTH OF BED.
Psor. *673*.

HYPERAESTHESIA IN ACUTE CONDITIONS, FOLLOWED BY ANAESTHESIA.
Plumbum. *665*.

REPEATED OUTBREAKS OF PUSTULES.
Psor. *676*.

ABNORMAL TENDENCY TO SKIN DISEASES.
Psor. *678*.

BLISTERS, WITH INTOLERABLE BURNING AND ITCHING.
Ran. b. *699*, Rhus. *715*.

EXCORIATED BY ACRID DISCHARGES ANYWHERE.
Sul. *791*.

DARK RED SWELLINGS.
Tarent. *799*.

SKIN AFFECTIONS OF DIRTY FILTHY PEOPLE.
Sul. *792*.

LOOKS DIRTY (AND CANNOT BE WASHED CLEAN)
Psor. Thuja. *829*.

OLD SCARS CAUSING INDURATIONS AND LUMPS.
Graph. *396/7*. Dros. Sil. Graph. *398*.

PAPULES DEVELOPING INTO PUSTULES OR ULCERS.
Kali bich. *457*.

SUPPURATING TUBERCLES.
Kali bich. *461*.

DESQUAMATION OF EPIDERMIS.
Kali sul. *477*.

HYPERAESTHESIA — SCREAMS
 WHEN TOUCHED.
  Lach. Lac. can. *488.*

ECHYMOSES.
  Arn. then Ludum. *504* Ars. *97,*
  Canth. *194.*

< COLD WET WEATHER.
  Dulc. *363/4.*

< AT NIGHT.
  Mez. *546, 555.*

< HEAT OF BED OR FIRE.
  Mez. *546. 555.*

< TO TOUCH.
  Mez. *555.*

DANDRUFF.
  Nat. mur. *573.* Thuja. *828.*

SORE CORNERS TO MOUTH.
  Ant. crud. *52.*

HORNY EXCRESCENCIES.
  Ant. crud. *57.*

PIMPLES ON NOSE.
  Brom *138.* Cslc. p. *168.*

PIMPLES ON TONGUE.
  Brom. *138.*

PIMPLES ON FINGERS.
  Brom. *138.*

PIMPLES ON ARMS.
  Brom. *138.*

WITH SEVERE ITCHING OF SKIN.
  Ant. crud. *57,* Abrot. *1.* Chel.
  251.

PAPULES LIKE ACNE.
  Brom. *139,* Cicuta. *261.*

HARD PLACES ON NEWBORN.
  Camph. *176.*

COLD SWEAT ON SKIN.
  Colch. *302.*

ERYSIPELAS.
  Rhus. *709, 714. 716.* Ruta. *717.*
  Bellis. *127.* Bell. *129* Rhus.
  Canth. *195.* Cistus. *285.* Ipec.
  438. 443.

DRY, HOT.
  Ptelea. *680.* Stram. *775.*

DRY, HARSH.
  Alum. *39,* Calc. *163.* Psor. *675.*

MOTTLED.
  Ammon. carb. *45.*

SHINY SMOOTH RASH.
  Bell. *29.*

'MEASLY' RASH.
  Puls. (Ail. *29*).

ROUGH, CRACKS AND BLEEDS.
  Psor. *673.*

INTENSELY RED RASH.
  Stram. *775.*

DEEP REDNESS.
  Camph. *176.*

BLOATED.
  Caps. *204.*

FISSURED.
  Caust. *224.*

YELLOW. *Chel. 248. 251.* Crot.
  336.

DARK BROWN.
  Crot. *327.*

COLD AND DRY.
  Crot. *335, 337.*

COLD AND SWEATY.
  Lach. (Crot. *335. 337*) Ver.
  alb. *855.*

WITH THICK TOUGH LEATHERY
  CRUSTS.
  Mez. *556.*

PETECHIAE-LIKE PURPLE
SPOTS.
Arn. Phos. Crot. Ledum. *507.*

IMPETIGO.
Ant. tart. *59.* Ant crud. *57.*

ACNE AS RESULT OF
VACCINATION.
Thuja. *823.*

ACNE ROSACEA.
Caust. *227.*

ACNE DUE TO WET COLD.
Bellis *127.*

ACNE PUNCTATA.
Kali br. *466.*

ACNE PUSTULOSA.
Kali br. *466.*

PUSTULES, ON LEGS.
Thuja. *825.*

PUSTULES, VARIOLA-LIKE.
PAINFUL, JOIN TO FORM
ULCERS.
Sil. *754.*

PUSTULAR ERUPTIONS.
Cicuta *266,* Rhus. Thuja.
Variolinum. Chel. *251. Ant. tart.
60, 62, 66, 69.* Bell. *123.* Iris.
451, Kali bich. *460/1*

SIMILAR TO SMALL POX.
Ant tart. *62.*

SLEEP

SLEEPLESS:
from mental depression.
Thuja. *829.*
from effects of grief. Ign. *425.*

from effects of night watching.
Cocc. Colch. *305.*

from effects of mental activity.
Hyos. *414.* Nux. v. *609.*

from overexertion. Arn. (Kali
br. *462*).

from extreme weariness of
body and mind. Kali br. *462.*

from anxiety, fear. Acon. Kali
br. *462.*

from fear, terror. Ars. (Kali
br. *463*).

from Bright's disease. Kali br.
467.

from ebullition of blood. Puls.
685.

from excess mental and
physical excitement.
Coffea. *301.*

after re-vaccination. Thuja.
829.

NOT from tossing about.
Coffea. *300,* Ars. Hyos. *414.*

NOT from discomfort. Coffea
300.

NOT from pain. Coffea. *300*

with restlessness. Ledum. *506,*
Opium, *616.* Thuja. *829.*

with acuteness of hearing
Opium *613. 616.*

during teething. Kali br. *467.*

during whooping cough. Kali
br. *467.*

sleepy, but cannot sleep. Puls.
681, Cham. *241,* Cocc. *291.*
Opium. *616* Caul. *219. 230.*
Kreos. 480.

178

broken sleep. Cocc. (China. *257*) Ferr. *371*.

drowsy by day, sleepless at night. Ammon carb. *42*. Nitric ac. *593*.

POOR SLEEP AFTER MIDNIGHT.
Ars. *100*, Nitric ac. *593*.

WAKES EARLY AND CANNOT GET OFF AGAIN.
Bellis. *120*. Ferr. *371*. Nux. v. *609*.

LIGHT SLEEPER.
Acon. *10*.

RESTLESS.
Acon. *11*. Bell. *123*. Caul. *219*. Cina *280*, Glon. *391*. SI1. *755* Mur. ac. *563*. Lac can. *488*. Ledum. *506*.

WITH DREAMS.
Acon. *11*. Borax. *136*, Caps. *202*. Crot. *339*. Ign. *431*.

WITH MOUTH WIDE OPEN.
Ammon. carb. *45*.

STARTS UP IN FRIGHT IN HIS SLEEP.
Puls. *685*.

CHATTERS IN HIS SLEEP.
Puls. *685*.

VERY DEEPLY.
Agar. *24*. Cann. *183*. Con. *328*.

EXCESSIVE SLEEPINESS.
Cann. *183*, Caps. *202*. *204*. Phos. *647*, Plumbum. *669* Hyos. *414*. Nux. mosch. *597*. Iodum. Nux. mosch. *600*.

GREAT SLEEPINESS AFTER DINNER IN EVENING.
Nat. mur. *569*.

DROWSY DURING DAY, WAKEFUL AT NIGHT.
Sul. *791*.

DROWSY IN MORNING.
Phos ac. *638*.

DROWSY IN AFTERNOONS.
Staph. *764*.

DROWSY — DIFFICULT TO KEEP AWAKE.
Tereb. *813*. Ail. *26/7*, Chel. *249*.

SOPORIFIC, WITH SNORING.
Opium. *616*, Ign. *431*.

LOSS OF SLEEP AGGRAVATES ALL SYMPTOMS.
Cocc. *298*.

SLIGHTEST LOSS OF SLEEP AFFECTS HIM.
Cocc. *295*.

> AFTER SHORT SLEEP.
Camph. Phos. Sepia, Phos ac. *636*. Phos. *643*.

COMPLAINTS > FROM SLEEP.
Sepia. *747*.

GREAT SLEEPINESS DURING DAY.
Ant. crud. *54, 56*. Ant. tart, *63*. *68* Phos. *646*.

CHILD WILL NOT SLEEP IN THE DARK.
Stram. *775*.

CHILD SOON FALLS ASLEEP IN LIGHTED ROOM.
Stram. *775*.

CHILD SLEEPS IN KNEE-CHEST POSITION.
Med. (Aeth. *18*).

CHILD STARTS FROM SLEEP AS
   IF SMOTHERING.
   Ammon. carb. *45*, Cina *282*.

CHILD CHEWS AND SWALLOWS
   WHILE ASLEEP.
   Calc. *162*.

SCREAMING DURING SLEEP.
   Bell. *123/4* Borax *132*. *136*.

LAUGHING DURING . . .
   Hyos. *412*.

MOANING IN . .
   Cham. *241*.

WAKES IN FRIGHT WHEN JUST
   FALLING ASLEEP.
   Bell. *123*.

SLEEPS ON HER FACE.
   Med. Cina. Lac. can. *488*,
   Med. *528*.

GETTING ON AND LYING ON
   HANDS AND KNEES
   DURING . .
   Med. Cina. *281*.

FEELS SUFFOCATED AND
   OBLIGED TO SIT UP ALL
   NIGHT.
   Ant. tart. *69*.

WAKES AT 3–5 A.M., CANNOT
   SLEEP AGAIN.
   Sul. *791*.

< ON WAKING.
   Lach. Ant. tart. *62*. Ammon
   carb. *46*, *Crot. 337*.

< FOR WARMTH.
   Ant. tart. *68*.

WITH PERSPIRATION.
   Cicuta. *263*.

GRITTING ITS TEETH DURING . .
   Cina. *281*, Nat. phos. *576*.

JERKING IN . .
   Cina. *281*.

COUGHING IN . .
   Cina. *281*.

IN A COMA.
   Opium. *615*.

SLEEPLESS ON ACCOUNT OF
   FEELING OF SICKNESS.
   Ornithogalum. *619*.

WITH NIGHTMARES.
   Sul. *791*.

SMALLPOX
   Thuja. *819*.

SPASMS
OF TEETHING BABIES.
   Bell. *119*

OF THROAT > COLD.
   Lach (Lyc. *522*)

OF THROAT > WARM.
   Lyc. *522*.

OF THROAT, SOMETIMES >
   WARM DRINKS.
   Lyc. *522*.

OF CIRCULAR MUSCLES. E.G. OF
   BILE DUCT.
   Bell. *119*.

OF ALL HOLLOW MUSCULAR
   ORGANS.
   Vib. *863*.

BEGINS IN FINGERS AND TOES,
   SPREAD AND BECOMES
   GENERAL.
   Cup. 343.

IN ARMS AND FINGERS.
   Cicuta. *264*.

VIOLENT.
Cicuta. *264*, Cocc. *296*.

TONIC AND CLONIC.
Cicuta. *265*, Pet. *629*.

HYSTERICAL.
Cimic. *274*.

LIKE ELECTRIC SHOCKS.
Cocc. *294*.

WITH IRREGULAR PAROXYSMS.
Cup. *342*.

WITH SYMPTOMS IN GROUPS.
Cup. *342*.

FROM EMOTIONAL CAUSES.
Kali br. *406*, Opium. *616*.

TETANIC SPASMS.
Phyt. *652*.

TETANIC SPASMS. FROM
SWALLOWING TOBACCO.
Ipec. *446*.

SPASMODIC BREATHING.
Cup. *343*.

WITH THUMBS CLENCHED.
Cup *346*.

AFTER VEXATION OR FRIGHT.
Cup. *346*, Ign. *426*.

> COLD WATER.
Cup. *343*.

IN WHOOPING COUGH.
Cup. 342.

FROM SLIGHTEST TOUCH
Cicuta *263*, Nux. v. *607*.

IN CONVULSIONS.
Bell. *119*. Cicuta *261*, Ipec.
443, Phyt. *652*.

PUERPERAL SPASMS.
Hyos. *414*.

SPASMODIC STAMMERING.
Mag. phos. *525*.

SPASMODIC STAMMERING WITH
CONSTRICTION OF THROAT.
Mag. phos. *525*.

WITH ACID SYMPTOMS.
Nat. phos. *576*.

ON SEEING WATER.
Lyssin, Tereb. *814*.

ON SEEING A BRIGHT OBJECT.
Tereb. *814*.

ON ATTEMPTING TO URINATE.
Tereb. *814*.

< LEFT SIDE.
Ipec. *443*.

< ON WALKING.
Lach. *497*.

> FROM SHAKING THE PART
(E.G. A LEG)
Fluoric ac. Brom. *138/9*.

SPECIFICS
REMEDIES WHERE DRUG AND
DISEASE PICTURES COINCIDE.
Mez. *547*.

ANGINA.
Latrod (Canth *196*) (Crot.
332).

BLACKWATER FEVER.
Crot. *332*.

BLEEDING PILES.
Hypericum. *422*.

CYSTITIS.
Canth. *196*.

DYSENTERY.
Merc. cor. (Canth. *196*) (Crot
332).

181

GOUT.
Colch. *302.*

ORBITAL CELLULITIS.
Rhus. *710.*

PTOMAINE POISONING.
Arsenicum. (Crot. *332*).

SCARLET FEVER.
Bell. (Canth. *196*) (Crot. *332*)

STRAINS AND SPRAINS.
Rhus. *710.*

TINEA KERION.
Mez. (CM) *547.*

ULCERATION OF CORNEA IN CHILDREN.
Bacillinum. (Tub. *834*).

WRIST AND ANKLE SPRAINS.
Ruta *718/9.*

SPEECH
INCOHERENT.
Cann. *183.*

DIFFICULT.
Cocc. *290.*

SPHINCTERS
CONTRACTION.
Bell. *124.*

SPINE
BACKACHE:
with jerkings and trembling of limbs. Aga. *22.*

with flatulence, Colicy leucorrhea. Aesc. *14.*

with rectal symptoms. Aesc. *14.*

with sacral pains. Agar. *22.*

> passing urine. Lyc. *519.*

paralytic weaknesses with pain.
Cocc. *297.*

from below up. Con. *324.*

< caused by anger and indignation. Coloc. *314.*

cramp-like pains in region of kidneys. Caust. *229.*

PAIN IN:
small of back. Cocc. *293*, Kali carb. *473* Nat. mur, Sepia *738 743* Sul. *790.*

upper dorsal vertebrae. Cimic. *272.*

lumbar and sacral areas. Cimic. *273*, Cocc. *292*. Dulcl. *366.*

sacrum. Cina. *283*, Hyp. *419.*

across shoulders. Cann. *183.*

lumbo-sacral area < slightest movement. San. *735*, Ant. tart *68* Bry. *144.*

in spine or sacrum. Nux. mosch. *597.*

shoulder joint. Staph. *764.*

coccyx when sitting. Kali bich. *458.*

numbness in coccyx when sitting. Plat. *661.*

coccyx, painful. Sil. *753*, Sul. *790.*

coccyx – injuries to . . Hyp (Symphitum *794*).

coccyx. pain. Caust. *229*, Hyp. *418.*

INJURIES TO LUMBAR AREA.
Con. *323*. Hyp. (Symphitum *794*).

LANCINATIONS LIKE NEEDLES IN DORSAL SPINE.
Crot. casc. (Crot. *340*).

TEARING DOWNWARDS THROUGH WHOLE SPINE.
Cina. *283*.

ACHE IN MIDDLE OF SPINE.
Mur. ac. *565*.

UNABLE TO STOOP ON ACCOUNT OF PAIN.
Kali bich. *458, 460*.

PAIN:
< walking. Cocc. *283*. Kali carb. *473* > walking. Sepia *743*.

< motion. Aesc. *14*.

shooting up dorsal spine to occiput Pet. *633*. Phos. *643*.

violent, with opisthotonos. Nat. sul. *582*.

> heat. Mag. phos. *527*.

< touch. Lac. can. *488*.

< pressure. Lac. can. *488*.

shooting down to gluteal muscles or hips. Kali carb. *473*.

as if hot iron thrust into spine. Alum. *39*.

> STRAIGHTENING AND BENDING STIFFLY BACKWARDS.
Aeth. *20*.

> PRESSURE AGAINST SOMETHING HARD.
Sepia *742*.

UMBILICAL PAIN GOES THROUGH TO BACK.
Plat. *662*.

RHEUMATIC PAIN IN SHOULDER.
Sang. *729*.

NERVE PAINS IN SPINE.
Coloc. *314*.

DRAWING PAINS IN OR NEAR SPINE.
Caps. *202*.

SCAPULAE:
interscapular pains. Cicuta. *263*.

burning. Lyc. Phos. Sul. *782*. Phos. *643 646* Glon. *390*.

> warmth. Rhus. *710*.

< cold. Rhus. *710*.

icy cold between . . Sepia *743, 744*, Caps. *203*.

pain between . . Ars. *93*, Calc. *163*. Lyc. *515*. Phos. Kali bich Lyc. *519*.

pain in left scapula. Tub. *834*.

< lying down. Tub. *834*.

> warmth. Tub. *834*.

pain in left scapula when at rest. Coloc. *319*.

drawing sensation in right scapula. Coloc. *319*.

stitches in and between . . . Nitric ac. *592*.

CHILLINESS ALONG SPINE.
Gels. *386*, Mag. phos. *525*.

INFLAMMATIONS.
Canth. *195*.

BURNINGS:

> by heat. Ars. Picric ac. *655.*

< between scapulae. Phos. Kali br. Lyc. Picric ac. *655* Thuja *829.*

throbbing > rubbing. Phos. Picric ac. *655.*

< mental exertion. Picric ac. *655, 657.*

in lumbar area. Theridion, Picric ac. *655/7* Tereb. *810.*

least study causes burning along spine. Picric ac. *655.*

COLDNESS DOWN SPINE.
Picric ac. *657* Thuja. *829.*

SENSATION OF DAMP CLOTHES ON SPINE.
Tub. *839.*

PARALYTIC WEAKNESS.
Phos. ac. (Picric ac. *655*).

PARALYSIS FROM SOFTENING OF THE CHORD.
Picric ac. *655.*

SMALL OF BACK STIFF, BRUISED.
Rhus. *713.*

< moving about Rhus. *713.*

as if beaten. Ruta *721.*

FEELING OF CONGESTION.
Ver. vir. *860.*

DULL ACHE.
Aesc. *14.*

WEAK.
Aesc. *14,* Picric ac. *657.*

< MOVEMENT.
Kali carb. *473.*

> 3 A.M.
Kali carb. *473.*

< PRESSURE.
Theridion. *817.*

< LEAST NOISE.
Theridion. *817.*

LEAST JAR. THERIDION. *817.*

SITTING
Agar. *22.*

MOVEMENT.
Agar. *22.*

CEREBRO-SPINAL MENINGITIS.
Ferr. phos. *379,* Ipec. *441,* Ail. *27,* Cicuta Nat. sul. *582.* Cicuta. Ver. vir. *860 Cicuta 261, 265.*

PARAPLEGIA.
Cocc. *295.*

CONCUSSIONS OF, RESULTING IN PARAPLEGIA.
Con. *329.*

SPINAL SCLEROSIS.
Picric ac. *657.*

SPINAL CARIES.
Dros. *356/7.*

SCOLIOSIS AND T.B.
Dros *357*

DISEASES OF THE BONES OF . . .
Symphitum *796.*

LOCOMOTOR ATAXIA (DISEASE OF NERVOUS SYSTEM OF SPINAL CORD)
Plumbum *666* Cocc. *292, 294.* Con. *324.*

INCOORDINATION OF BRAIN AND SPINAL CORD.
Agar. *22.*

TUMOURS ABOUT VERTEBRAL COLUMN.
Tarent. *801.*

184

CURVATURE OF . .
Phos ac. *639*, Sul. *790*.

CONCUSSION.
Arn. Cicuta *261*, Hyp. *422/3*.

BACK BENT BACKWARDS LIKE
AN ARCH.
Cicuta *263*.

SUDDEN STIFFNESS OF BACK,
BENDING BACKWARDS.
Cham. *241*.

PSOAS ABSCESS FROM DISEASES
OF THE VERTEBRAE.
Symphitum. *797*.

STIFF NECK.
Phyt. *652*.
< movement. Bry. (Phyt.
652).
< on first movement. Rhus.
(Phyt. *752*).
< cold and draught. Phyt.
652.

FEELS AS IF BROKEN.
Nat. mur. *574*.

INTENSE ACHING FROM BRAIN
TO COCCYX.
Lac. can. *488*, Rhus. *708*.

DRAWING SENSATION IN LEFT
CERVICAL MUSCLES.
Coloc. *319*.

ILL EFFECTS FROM BRUISES AND
SHOCKS TO SPINE.
Con. *323*, Hyp. *416*.

PAINFUL AS RESULT OF COLD.
Dulc. *365*.

OLD JARS TO SPINE.
Glon. *390*.

SHOOTING PAINS FROM SEAT OF
INJURY.
Hyp. *419*.

< RISING FROM CHAIR.
Caust. *229*.

STIFF BACK.
Caust. *229*.

FATTY DEGENERATION OF . .
Picric ac. *655*.

SPLEEN
Dros. *360*.

CONGESTION OF SPLENIC
FEATURE.
Alum. *35*. Cean. *233*.

PAIN IN . .
Bellis *130*.

STITCHING PAINS
< MOVEMENT.
Bry. *144*

PAIN IN LEFT
HYPOCHONDRIUM.
Cean. *231* China. Chel. Berb.
Chin. sul. Con. (Cean. *231*).

< DRINKING ANYTHING COLD.
Cean. *233*.

WITH DYSPNOEIA.
Cean. *233*.

< ANY PRESSURE.
Cean. *233*.

CAUSING HEART TROUBLE.
Cean. *233*.

< COLD WEATHER.
Cean. *235*.

< LYING ON LEFT SIDE.
Cean *235*.

DROPSIES CURED BY SPLEEN
REMEDIES . .
Cean. *233*.

PAIN UNDER LEFT RIB.
Cean *233*.

SPLINTERS
see FIRST AID.

STAMMERING
Caust *224*.

STINGS
see FIRST AID

STOMACH
GASTRALGIA.
Ptelea. *679*.

of pregnancy. Pet. *629*.

when stomach is empty. Pet. *629*.

GASTRITIS.
Kali bich. *456*.

with constant vomiting. Ipec. *441*.

with blinding headaches. Caust. Nat. mur. Iris. v. Psor. Kali bich. *456*.

acidic. Nat. phos. *576*.

< eating or drinking. Kali bich. *457*.

DYSPEPSIA, WITH HEADACHE.
Kali bich. *456*.

with putrid eructations. Sal. ac. *725*.

STOMACHACHE.
Carbo v. *212*. Kali bich. *454*. Nat. phos. *576*, Sul. *788*.

GASTRIC DERANGEMENTS DUE
TO OVEREATING.
Ant. crud. *56*.

INDIGESTION.
Borax. *132*.

PYLORUS – SPASMODIC
CONTRACTION.
Ornithogalum. *617*. *619*.

constricted. Crot. *336*.

ECCHYMOSIS OF STOMACH
MUCOUS MEMBRANES.
Sal. ac. *724*. Tereb. *810*.

HAEMORRHAGES IN . .
Sal. ac. 725.

DISCOMFORT IN
HYPOGASTRIUM.
Cycl. *350*.

CONGESTION.
Ver. vir. *860*.

FEELING AS IF:
lime were slaking in . . Caust. *224*.

something alive in . . Ver. alb. *856*.

stomach were tightly drawn against the spine. Plumb. Plat. Ver. Vir. *862*.

there were a lump in . . Bry. San. *734*.

the stomach were like a leather bag. Kali bich. *455*.

food lay in the stomach like a load. Kali bich. *455*. *459*.

GURGLING IN STOMACH.
Phos. (Cup. *344*) Cycl. *350*. Ign. *430*.

CANNOT BEAR CLOTHES
AROUND . . .
Crot. *336* Lyc. *517*, Lach.
(Crot *339*) Crot. casc. (Crot.
339).

PIT OF STOMACH:
pinching on deep breathing.
Caust. *227*.

constriction, tension in . .
Chel. *250* Mez. *554*.

apprehension in . . Lyc. *516*,
Calc. Kali c. Phos. Mez. *556*.

throbbing in . . Cicuta *262*.

crawling at . . Alum. *37*.

spasms from sternum to . .
Iris. *452*.

SPASMS IN . .
Cocc. *296*, Iris. *452*. Mag.
phos. *524*.

PAIN IN ILEO-CAECAL REGION.
< TOUCH < MOTION.
Plumbum. *670*.

CRAMP IN . .
Caust *227*. Crot. *336*, Mag.
phos. *525*.

SINKING FEELING IN . .
Cimic. *275*.

GNAWING SENSATION IN . . . AS
FROM HUNGER.
Cina. *283*.

SICK FEELING IN . .
Ipec. *445*.

ROUND ULCER IN . .
Kali bich. *460*.
> eating or drinking with
reappearance of rheumatic
pains. Kali bich. *460*.

ULCER OF . . .
Mez. *552*, Nat. phos. *576*,
Ornithogalum. *619*.

PRESSURE IN . .
Lyc. *517*.

DERANGED FROM EATING EGGS.
Colch. *308*.

FEELS FLABBY.
Ign. *430*.

PAIN:
in small spot by xyphoid. Kali
bich. *454*.

alternating with pain in limbs.
Kali bich. *460*.

in hard spot at left of . . Kreos
479.

pressive. Acon. *10*, Cicuta,
262, Nux. v. *605*.

< motion. Bry. *143*.

tensive. Acon. *10*.

burning. Ail. *28*, Ant. crud. *55*,
Ars. *94*. Cicuta *262*. Colch. *304*
Ars. *99*. Carbo v. *209, 211*,
Mez. *553*.

as from fullness, without
fullness. Ant. crud. *55*.

with distended but not hard
abdomen. Ant. crud. *55*.

griping and cutting < motion.
Bry. *143*, Ptelea *680*.

on stretching. Ammon. carb.
42.

stitching < motion. Bry. *144*.

cutting constricting. Graph.
399 < motion. Bry. *143*.

only when stomach is empty.
Anac (200C) *50*.

> eating. Anac. *50*. Graph.
399, Chel. Pet. *630*.

> after digestion process is
over. Nux. v. Anac. *50*.

< 2–3 hours after meals. Nux.
v. Anac. *50*.

clutching, cramping and
digging. Coloc. *316* >
pressure. Coloc. *316*.

violent. Con. *329*, Iris. *451*,
Nux. v. *605*.

BLOATED.
Lyc. *517*, Aeth. *17*, Arg. nit.
80, Ail. *28*. Carbo v. *209*,
Graph. *398*. Ant crud. *55*. Ars.
94. Cicuta. *262*.

AS IF HANGING.
Abrot. *2*. Ipec. *445*.

AS IF SWIMMING IN WATER.
Abrot. *2*.

TENSION. > DRINKING MILK.
Ruta. *720*.

> DRINKING VERY HOT
WATER.
Pyrogen. *690*.

< PRESSURE.
San. *734*.

< JAR.
San. *734*.

> EXTERNAL PRESSURE.
Ammon. carb. *43*.

PAIN IN LOWER PART OF . .
Ver. vir. *862*.

FOOD LIES IN STOMACH LIKE A
LOAD.
Kali bich. *455*. *459*.

FEELING OF FULLNESS.
Puls. Kali sul. *475*.

FEELING OF EMPTINESS.
Mur. ac. *565*, Ptelea. *680*.

MALIGNANT ULCERATION OF . .
Ornithogalum. *619*.

INDIGESTION WITH EXCESSIVE
ERUCTATIONS OF WIND.
Ornithogalum. *619*.

ACID STOMACH.
Nat. phos. *575*.

SENSATION OF PINS IN . .
Med. *534*.

'ALL-GONE' SENSATION.
Sepia. *747*.

GRIPING IN EPIGASTRIUM.
Cocc. *296*. Lyc. *517*.

INFLAMMATION OF . .
Hyos. *414*.

PULSATIONS IN . .
Asaf. *103*.

SWOLLEN.
Calc. *154, 161*. Carbo v. *212*.
Dulc. *363*.

SENSATION OF COLD WATER
IN . .
Caps. *204*.

FLATUS IN . .
Carbo v. *212*.

COLDNESS IN . .
Carbo v. *207*, Cocc. *298*,
Colch. *304*, Crot. *388* Kali
bich. *459* Abrot. *2*. Caps. *201*.

WEAK.
Caps. *204*.

AS IF STONE IN . .
Bry. *149* Cham. *240*.

ALL SYMPTOMS CENTRE
ROUND . . .
Ant. crud. 56.

STOMATITIS

INFLAMMATION OF MUCOUS
MEMBRANE OF THE MOUTH.
see MOUTH.

STOOLS

PAINFUL DURING AND AFTER.
Nitric ac. Aesc. *14*. Alum *36*.
Colch. *307*. Nat. mur. *572*.

PAINFUL SOME HOURS AFTER
STOOL.
Aesc. *14*. Ratanhia. *Nitric ac.*
588.

WITH SPASMODIC PAIN OF
SPHINCTER AFTER STOOL.
Colch. *305, 307*.

PASSED WITH GREAT
EXERTION.
Hepar. *405*, Plat. *660*, Nux.
mosch. *599*.

PASSED WITH GREAT PAIN.
Med. *535*. Hepar. *405*.

PAINLESS.
Psor. *677*.

INTOLERABLE PAIN DURING
AND AFTER.
Paeonia. *624*.

PAIN IN PERINEUM WHILE AT
STOOL.
San. *734. 737*.

SUPPRESSED.
Stramm. *775*.

PASSES ONLY WHEN LEANING
BACK.
Med. *531, 535*.

CAN ONLY PASS WHEN
STANDING.
Alum. *38*.

PASSES BETTER WHEN
STANDING.
Caust. *224. 228*.

PERINEUM SORE AND BURNING
AFTER STOOL.
Nitric ac. San. *734*.

TENESMUS.
Caps. *201*, Kali bich. *458*.

AFTER A DRINK, MUST GO TO
STOOL.
Caps. *203*.

INABILITY TO STRAIN DUE TO
PARALYTIC WEAKNESS OF
MUSCLES.
Con. *323*.

WITH PROTRUSION OF
STOMACH.
Ant. crud. *55*.

WITH BLACK BLOOD.
Ant. crud. *55*.

WITH PARTLY SOLID, PARTLY
fluid STOOLS.
Ant. crud. *56*.

COLIC BEFORE.
Ant. tart. *67*, Nitric ac. *591*.

LONG INTERVALS BETWEEN
STOOLS.
Arn. 89.

WITH PUS.
Calc. p. *168*.

FLATULENT.
Olean. Aloe. Psor. *674*.

FEEL FULL OF JAGGED
PARTICLES.
San. *734*.

INVOLUNTARY:
Phos ac. *638*, San. *734*, Bapt.
115. Aloe. Caust. *224*. Hyos.
413/4.

after fright. Opium. *614*. *616*.

almost . . . Psor. *677*.

during sleep. Arn. *89*.

from excitement. Hyos. *411*.

while urinating. Hyos. *415*.

while straining to urinate.
Mur. ac. *504*.

from paralysis of sphincter.
Hyos. *415*.

AFRAID TO STRAIN BECAUSE
'SOMETHING WILL BREAK'
Apic. *75*.

GREAT AND URGENT DESIRE.
Anac. *48*. *51*. Sul. Psor. *674*.

FREQUENT DESIRE.
Lil. tig. *509*. Nux. v. *606*.
Abrot. *2*. Nux. v. Anac. *51*.
Ign *431*.

FREQUENT URGING WITH
SCANTY STOOLS.
Hyos. *411*. Puls. *684*. Nux. v.
606. Plat. *661*.

MUST GO TO STOOL AFTER
EATING.
Brom. *141*. San. *734*.

HURRIED EARLY MORNING
STOOLS.
Sul. *783*. *788*.

IN MORNING AFTER RISING.
Nat. sul. *583*.

FREQUENT INEFFECTUAL
EFFORTS TO STOOL.
Sil. *753*, *Nux v*. *606*. Caust. *226*

Nitric ac. *591*. Ign. *430*. Sepia
(Lach. *496*.) Merc. *542*.

VIOLENT URGING.
Agar. *22*, Ant. crud. *55*,
Cicuta. *269*. Colch. *307*, Hyos.
414, Ign. *430*. Graph. *399*.
Hepar. *405*. Plat. *661*.

AFTER STOOL, FEELING OF
SOME REMAINING BEHIND.
Nux v. *606*.

hungry. Pet. *631/2*.

weakness and palpitation.
Con. *328*.

thirst. Caps. *201*, *203*.

burning. Bry. *149*.

tired. Merc. *544*.

STOOLS:
like coffee grounds. Tereb.
810.

hard dry. Opium. *616*, Phos.
642, Plumbum. *666*, *668*. Tub.
837.

hard, dry, knotty. Aesc. *14*.
Alum. *36*, Ant. crud. *54*, Bry.
145, *148*, Graph. *399*. Collin.
311. Caust. *224*. Mez. *553*.

dry faecal matter. Opium.
(Collin. *313*).

dry faecal matter – light
coloured. Collin. *313*.

loose. Calc. p. *168*, Phos. *642*.

slimy. Calc. p. *168*, Merc. *538*.

mushy. Calc. p. *168*.

soft. Nux. mosch. *596*.

but difficult to expel. Alum.
China. Nux. mosch.
Psor. *674*. San. *734*.

Alum. *36*. Calc. p. *168*.
Hepar. *405*.

gelatinous. Colch. *307*.

bloody. Colch. *307*, Crot. *336*.
Ferr. phos. *379, 380* Nitric ac.
591 Merc. *538*. *543*.

sluggish. Collin. *311*. Nux.
mosch. *597*.

cool. Con. *330*.

undigested. Ferr. *370*. Graph.
399. Nux. mosch. *597*.

lumpy. Graph. *399*.

lumpy and soft. Lyc. *518*.

sudden gushing, noisy.
spluttering. Nat. sul. *583*.

of mucous. Caps. *201*. Collin.
311. Graph. *399*.

'bashful', slipping back when
almost voided. Sil. *751*. *755*,
Opium, Sil. Lac. d. Nat. mur.
Thuja. San. *732*. Sil. Thuja.
San. *734*.

'never get done' sensation.
Merc. cor. Merc. *538*. Nux. v.
606.

NO TWO STOOLS ALIKE.
Puls. (Kali sul. *476*) San. *737*.

DIARRHOEIA-LIKE
Kali bich. *458*.

HARD, EVACUATED WITH
GREAT EXERTION.
Sil. *751*. *753*. Nat. mur. *573*
Nitric ac *592*. San. *734*.

DIARRHOEIC – SMELL OF
ROTTEN EGGS.
Psor. *673*.

VERY OFFENSIVE.
Calc. p. *168*. Pod. (Cup. *344*).
Sil. *751*. Graph. *399*. Psor. *676/
7*.

DARK BROWN.
Psor. *676*.

GREEN.
Nat. phos. *576*.

GREY.
Chel. *247*, Phos. ac. *638*. Phos.
645.

LIGHT COLOURED. LUMPY.
Collin. *311*.

CLAY COLOURED.
Hepar. *405*.

WHITE.
Acon. *10*. Aesc. *14*. Calc. *153*.
Calc. p. *168*. Puls *684*.

PROFUSE GREENISH.
Asaf. *103*. Calc. p. *168*. *170*
Ipec. *443*.

YELLOW.
Borax. *135*. Chel. *247*. *250*.
Puls. *684*. San. *734*.

BLACK FAECAL.
Brom. *141*. Cicuta. *269*. Collin.
311. Crot. *333*. Med. *535*.

GREEN, SLIMY, ACRID.
Merc. *543*.

VERY HOT.
Calc. p. *168*.

SOUR.
Calc. *153*. *157*. Nat. phos. *576*.

FETID.
Bapt. *115*. Cret. *336*. Graph.
395, 399 Merc. *537*.

VERY LIQUID.
Ant. crud. *53*. Asaf. *102*. Calc.
161. Calc. p. *168*. Colch. *309*
Ferr. phos. *379*, Graph. *395,
399*. Psor. *677*, Iris. *450*.

ACRID AND EXCORIATING.
Ammon. carb. *45*, Lyc. Calc.
153.

ODOUR, STRONG, LONG
LASTING.
San. *732*.

PUTRID, PENETRATING ODOUR.
Bapt. *113*. Calc. *157*, Graph.
395.

DYSENTERIC.
Bapt. *114*. Collin. *311*.

DISGUSTING ODOUR.
Asaf. *102/3*. Graph. *399*. Merc.
537.

MEMBRANOUS.
Brom. *141*. Canth. *197*.

STRABISMUS
SQUINTING.   see EYES.

STRANGURY
INFLAMMATION OF KIDNEYS,
BLADDER OR URINARY
PASSAGES RESULTING IN
CONSTANT DESIRE TO PASS
WATER.   see BLADDER.

STRYCHNINE
POISONING
Cham. *243*.

STUPOR
Ail. *28. 29*. Bell. *124*.

WITH INVOLUNTARY
DISCHARGE OF FAECES.
Arn. *88*.

WITH CONVULSIONS.
Opium. *616*.

WITH SLEEPING.
Tereb. *810*.

FROM CONCUSSION.
Arn. *88*.

MIND GONE, STATE OF STUPOR.
Bapt. *113*.

FALLS ASLEEP WHILE BEING
SPOKEN TO.
Bapt. *115*.

FALLS ASLEEP WHILE
ANSWERING.
Bapt. *115*.

DURING SCARLET FEVER.
Bapt. *114*.

DELIRIOUS STUPOR.
Bapt. *115*.

INSENSIBILITY.
Nux. mosch. *596*. Opium. *616*.

SUBSULTUS
TWITCHING.
Mez. *556*. Hyos. *414*.

SUICIDE
see MENTALS.

SUNSTROKE
Bel. *117*. Glon. *390*.

SWEAT
PROFUSE.
Bell. *125*. Bry. *150*. Calc. *153/4
156 159* Ferr. phos. *380*. Sil.

Hepar. *401*. Merc. *537*. Cann.
183. Dulc. *364*. Tub. *837*. Merc
538/9. 543, Opium. *615/6*. Sal.
ac. *725*. Psor. *676*. Sepia *738*.
Sil. *755*. Agar. *26*.

PROFUSE, WITHOUT RELIEF.
Merc. *539*. Phos. *647*.

PROFUSE, AFTER ACUTE
DISEASES, BRINGING RELIEF.
Psor. *672*.

PROFUSE ON SLIGHTEST
EXERCISE.
Psor. *677*.

PROFUSE, DURING SLEEP, DAY
OR NIGHT.
Con. *323*. (reverse Sambucus.
San. *732*. Con. *325)*.

PROFUSE ON AFFECTED PARTS.
Ambra. Merc. Rhus. Ant.
tart. (Con. *326)*.

CONSTANT.
Colch. *306*.

CONSTANT ON CLOSING EYES.
Calc. Carb. an. Thuja. Bry.
Lach. Con. *326/7 329*. San. *736*.

WITH GREAT THIRST.
China 260.

WITH SMARTING SENSATION IN
SKIN.
Cham. *242*.

WITH VOMITING.
Camph. *176*.

WITH PALPITATION.
Lach. (Con. *326)*.

WITH ITCHING ON WAKING.
Ledum. *506*.

SLIGHT, OVER WHOLE BODY.
Acon. *11*.

LACK OF . . .
Nux. mosch. *597*.

PARTIAL SWEATS.
Calc. *163*.

ONLY ON COVERED PARTS.
Bell. *125*, Cham. *242*.

NO SWEAT ON COVERED
PARTS.
Thuja. (Con. *326)*.

ONLY ON UNCOVERED PARTS.
Thuja (Bell *125*) (Camph.
176) (Cham. *242*) (Puls. *683*)
Thuja 820.

CANNOT BEAR TO BE
UNCOVERED DURING SWEAT.
Aeth. *20*.

DEBILITY FROM PROFUSE
SWEATS.
China. *255*.

COLD SWEATS.
Carbo. v. *207*. Hepar. *407*.
Ver. alb. *853 855*. San. *735*.
Phos. ac. *635*. Ver. vir. *862*.

on feet and legs. Sepia. Calc.
156. 158. Pyrogen., *695*. Colch.
306. Hepar (Calc. s. *172*)
Camph. *176*. Ver. alb. (xv).

while eating. Merc. (Con.
326).

on arms and hands. Phos. ac.
635.

cold, clammy. Ver. vir. *860/1*.

FOOT SWEATS.
Plumbum. *670*, Sal. ac. *725*.
San. *732/3*, Baryta carb. Sil.
754/5.

with soreness between toes.
Graph. Bar. c. Zinc.

suppressed. Sil. *757*.

offensive. Nitric ac. *586. 588*.
Pet. *631*.

ONE-SIDED SWEAT.
Bar. c. Chin. Nux. v. Phos.
Pet. Sul. Thuja. Puls *683*.
Puls. (Kali sul. *476*).

ONE-SIDED SWEATS OF FACE.
Puls. *683*.

CLAMMY.
Pyrogen *695*, Tereb. *813*.

STICKY.
Cann. *183*.

STAINS LINEN YELLOW.
Tub. *837*.

WITH RAVENOUS HUNGER.
Phos *647*.

ALL OVER AFTER A MEAL.
Nitric ac. *591*.

**COMPLAINTS INCREASE WITH
SWEATS.**
Tilia. Merc. *539. 543*.

HUNGRY DURING SWEATS.
San. *736*.

**SUCCESSION OF CHILL, HEAT,
SWEAT.**
China. *256*.

ON BEING COVERED.
China. *260*, San. *736*.

> ON WAKING.
Chel. *251*.

< WALKING IN OPEN AIR.
Rhod. *705*.

**ON MAKING ANY MOTION,
SWEAT DISAPPEARS AND
HEAT COMES ON.**
Lyc. (Con. *326*).

ON PAINFUL PARTS.
Kali c. (Con. *326*).

ONLY WHILE AWAKE.
Sepia. Sambucus (Con. *326*).

FROM MUSIC.
Tarent. (Con. *326*).

SMELLING OF SULPHUR.
Phos. *644*.

SOUR.
Bry. *150*. Cham. *242*. Hepar.
407. Nat. phos. *475*.

BLOODY.
Lach. Nux mosch. (Con. *326*).
Crot. *335*.

OFFENSIVE.
Dulc. *364, 366*. Hepar. *406*.
407. Med. *537*. Sil. *751*. Merc.
543. Pet. *631*.

ON HANDS.
Nitric ac. *586*. Calc. *163*.

ON NECK, CHEST.
Calc. *163*.

ON FOREHEAD.
Carbo v. *212*.

ON HEAD AT NIGHT.
Calc. Merc. Sil. Sepia *743*, Sil.
755. Calc Sil. (Con. *326*).

ON LEGS.
Tereb. *813*.

**ON HAND AND FEET, WARM
SWEATS.**
Ledum. *506*.

HOT SWEAT ON HEAD.
Cham. *237*. Con. *329*. Calc.
carb. (Ferr. phos. *375*).

ON HEAD.
Calc. 156. 159. Calc. p. *170*.
San. *737*. Sepia. *743*.

LIKE GARLIC IN ARMPITS.
  Sul. *790.*

SWEET STRONG PUNGENT.
  Thuja. *820.*

ODOUR OF SPICE.
  Rhod. *705.*

OFFENSIVE, CARRION-LIKE.
  Pyrogen. *694.*

ON SLIGHTEST MOTION.
  Hepar. *406.* Phos. *647.* Agar.
  26.

ON PAINFUL PARTS.
  Kali carb. *469.*

SWEATS, BUT CANNOT BEAR TO
  BE COVERED.
  Ledum. *501.*

< HEAT OF BED.
  Ledum. *506.*

SWEAT THAT ATTRACTS FLIES.
  Caladium (Con. *326*).

INNER CONGESTION,
  EXTREMITIES COLD PROFUSE
  SWEAT.
  Calc. 158.

WITHOUT HEAT.
  Calc. *154.*

WHEN COLD.
  Calc. *154,* Cistus *287.*

AXILLARY SWEATS.
  Sil. (Hepar. *401*).

OFFENSIVE.
  Nitric ac. *588.*

WHEN WALKING.
  Agar. *26.*

< 3 A.M.
  Bry. *150.*

< 4–6 A.M.
  Ferr. phos. *380.*

SWELLING
EVERYTHING PUFFY.
  Carbo v. *207.*

SYPHILIS
  Mez. *546, 556.* Morb. *558.*
  Nitric ac. *588.*

T

TEETH
PAIN:
  after drinking anything warm.
  Cham. *239.*

  on extraction of teeth. *Arn.*
  239.

  in teeth. Arg. nit. *80.* Coloc.
  318. Glon. *389.*

  in hollow teeth. Ant. crud. *53.*

  toothache – neuralgic. > cold
  water in mouth. Coffea *300.*

    rheumatic. Ant. tart. *67.*

    throbbing. Caust. *227,* Hyp.
    423.

    caused by caries. Kreos.
    478, 481

    at 4 p.m. Lyc. *515.*

    < any solids or liquids.
    Staph. *761.*

    < cold. Calc. *160.*
    Theridion. *816.*

    > cold. Ferr. phos. *350.*

    twitching pain in hollow
    teeth. Mez. *554.*

  drawing pain. Bry. *148.*

  < 3 a.m. Bry. *148.*

> lying on painful cheek. Bry. *148*.

< at night. Ant. crud. *53*, Cham. *239*.

< after eating. Ant. crud. *53*. Arg. nit. *80*.

> walking in open air. Ant. crud. *53*. Calc. *160*.

stitching and tearing. Caust. *227*.

after drinking anything warm. Cham. *239*.

< talking. Cham. *239*.

< in open air. Cham. *239*.

> heat or hot liquids. Mag. phos. *524*.

violent at night. Merc. *542, 545*.

< during menstruation or pregnancy. Cham. *239*.

< from least draught. Sul. *788*, from washing with cold water. Sul. *788*.

LOOSE.
Carb. v. *212*. Merc. *541*. Nux. mosch. *597*.

CHATTERING.
Viscum. *868*.

SORDES (FILTH) ON TEETH.
Bapt. *115*. Caust. *217*. Hyos. *414*.

TEETH FEEL TOO LONG.
Cham. *239*.

DENTITION:
degeneration of teeth during . . . Kreos. *481*.

vomiting during . . . Calc. *161*.

diarrhoeia during . . . Calc. *161*.

screaming at night during . . . Kreos. *481*.

difficult. Calc. *160. 162*. Kreos. *482*.

slow. Calc. p. *166*.

delayed. Calc. *153*. Calc. p. *169*.

catarrhal hyperaemia during . . . Ant. tart. *67*.

CHILLY FEELING THROUGH TEETH . . .
Ant. tart. *67*.

CONVULSIVE GRINDING OF . . .
Coffea. *300*.

DECAY IN TEETH AS SOON AS ERUPTED.
Kreos *478*. Mez. *553*.

BAD ODOUR FROM DECAYED TEETH.
Kreos. *478*

CHOLERA INFANTUM AS RESULT OF PAINFUL DENTITION.
Kreos. *483*.

LOOSE WHEN CHEWING.
Nitric ac. *591*.

IRRESISTIBLE DESIRE TO BITE TEETH TOGETHER.
Phyt. *652/3*.

GRINDING OF TEETH.
Plumbum. *670*.

IF BLACK ON ERUPTION.
Staph. *761*.

IF FIRST TEETH DECAY QUICKLY.
Kreos. Staph. *761*.

TURN BLACK.
Staph. *762.*

TEMPERATURE

ALWAYS COLD.
Ars. *95*, Caps. *202*, Colch. *308.*
Ledum *502.* Nux v. *604.*

FREQUENTLY CHILLY.
Camph. *176.*

CHILLY AFTER EVERY DRINK.
Caps. *202.*

COLD, YET WANTS TO BE
FANNED.
Carbo v. *207.*

COLD, YET > FROM COLD.
Ledum. *501.* Nat. mur. (Phos.
641).

> WHEN COLD.
Iod. Puls. Lach. Nat. mur. Sul.
(Lyc. *521*).

< FROM COLD.
Sepia. Phos. *641.*

CHILLY ON SLIGHTEST
MOVEMENT.
Nux. v. *604. 608.*

CHILLY ON SLIGHTEST
EXPOSURE TO AIR OR
DRAUGHTS.
Nux. v. *604. 608.*

COLD, YET NO BETTER FROM
WARMTH.
Nux v. *608.*

< FROM DRAUGHTS.
Bell. *119.*

WANTS TO BE UNCOVERED.
Sul. Opium. *614.*

HIGH.
Bell. *117.*

BURNINGS RELIEVED BY HEAT.
Ars. *94.* Camph. *175.*

> WARMTH.
Cimic. *271.* Cistus. *288.*

EXTERNALLY WARM —
INTOLERABLE.
Ign. *431.*

EXTERNALLY WARM —
WITHOUT INTERNAL HEAT.
Ign. *431.*

< GETTING WARM IN BED.
Ledum. *502.* Merc. *529.*

> GETTING WARM IN BED.
Lyc. *521.* Ars. (Merc. *539*).

GREAT HEAT, YET GETS CHILLY
ON SLIGHTEST MOVEMENT OR
ON UNCOVERING.
Nux. v. *608.*

< HEAT.
Apis. *74.* Iodum. Brom. *138.
140.*

> PUTTING FEET IN COLD
WATER.
Puls. Ledum. *503.*

CANNOT BEAR HEAT.
Glon. Bell. *117.*

INTENSE HEAT.
Bell. *118.*

TENESMUS

CONSTANT SENSE OF WEIGHT
IN LOWER BOWEL, DESIRE TO
GO TO STOOL. see BLADDER
and STOOL.

TETANUS
Anac. *50.* Cocc. *294.* Hyp. *418.*
Ipec. *440.*

**AFTER PUNCTURED WOUNDS –
TO PREVENT TETANUS.**
Ledum *503*.
as result of . . Hyp. (Ledum
503).

**CONTRACTION OF JAWS LIKE
LOCKJAW.**
Tereb. *811* Nux v. *608*.
Theridion. *816*.

WITH DEATHLY COLDNESS.
Camph. (Phyt. *652*).

**WITH DRAWING UP CORNERS
OF MOUTH.**
Strychnia. Phyt. *652*.

TETANIC CONVULSIONS.
Ver. vir. *860*.

THIRST
THIRSTY:
Cocc. *296*. Mez. *531*. Merc.
(Nux mosch. *599*) Acon. *9*
Phos. (Ail. *29*) China. Bapt.
114. Caps. *204*. Cham. *240*.
for cold drinks. Rhus. *711*.
for acids. Cham. *240*.
during sweating. Ars. *96*.
China. *260*.
violent. Stram. *777*.
especially for beer. Cocc. *298*.
at night during sweat. Coffea.
301.
after heat and during sweat.
Coffea. *301*.
during chill. Ign. *425/6 428*.
Nat. mur. *570*.

for something very cold. Nat.
sul. *584*.
during evening. Cycl. *350*.
but eats little. Sul. *788*.
intense. Ant. c. rud. *53, 55*
Ant. tart. *66*, Bell. *124*. Bry.
148.½ Caust. *227*. Merc. *538*.
Nat mur. *572*. Stram. *774*.
Opium. *616* Tarent. *800*,
Cham. *242*. Merc. *537* Ars. *93*.
99. Bry. *149*. *150* Cham. *237*.
Crot. *336*.
for cold milk. Phos ac. *638*.
with dry throat. Rhus. *712*.
but dreads water. Stram. *770*.
with hunger. Ver. alb. *854*.
for very cold drinks. Ver. alb.
854.

THIRSTLESS:
Aeth. *18*. Ant. tart. *64. 66*.
Apis. *73*. Cina. *282*.
in fever. Puls. (Kali sul. *476*)
Nat. mur. *570*.
in chill. Puls (Kali sul. *476*)
Nux. mosch. *598*.
even with dry mouth. Nux.
mosch. *596, 598*. Puls. *686*.
during fever. Ign. *428*.
during day. Cycl. *350*. Colch.
307. Ipec. *441*.

**SHIVERING AFTER EVERY
DRINK.**
Cap. *201. 203/4*.

**SWALLOW OF COLD WATER
RELIEVES SPASMS.**
Caust. *227*.

THROAT

SORE.

Nux. v. *604*. Phyt. *654*. Phos. (Ail *29*) Calc. P. *166* Caps. *200* Ign. *430*. Ledum. *505*.

> swallowing. Ign. *425*. *428*.

mainly during menses. Lac. can. *488*.

from inhaling cold air. Cistus. *286*.

tender and sore on swallowing. Ail. *27*. Allium *32*. Caps. *200* Nitric ac. *591*.

as result of cold. Dulc. *365*.

BURNING.

Sul. *782*. Tereb. *810*. Mez. *552*, Paeonia. *622*. Sal. ac. *724* Caps. *200*. Caust. *227*, Cistus *286* Iris. *450* Acon. *9*. Aesc. *15* Apis. *74*. Bell. *118*. Canth. *197*.

LIVID.

Ail. *28*. Caps. *200*.

TICKLING.

Cham. *241*, Cistus. *286*. Iod. *434*.

IN TRACHEA WITH VIOLENT SNEEZING.

Caps. *203*.

PAIN EXTENDS TO RIGHT EAR.

Allium. *32*.

WITH PURPLE PATCHES.

Ail. *28*.

OEDAMATEOUS.

Ail. *28*. Apis. *74*.

ULCERATED.

Ail. *28*, Aur. *110*. Ferr. Bell. Phos. *380* Lach. *493, 498*.

DRY.

Acon. *11*. Aesc. *15*, Ail. *27*. Caps. *202*. Puls. *684*. Caust. *227* Cistus. *286*. Bell. (Crot. *332*). Lac. can. *487*. *490* Merc. *542*. Pet. *633*. Puls. *684*. Stram. *774*, Sul. *788*.

CONSTRICTED.

Acon. *11*. Chel. *250*, Cicuta *264*. Mez. *554*.

SPASMODIC CONSTRICTIONS

Con. *328*. Hyos. *415*. Mag. phos. *525*. Stram. *774* Crot. *336*. Gels. *385*. Glon. *390*. Plumbum. *668*.

PAIN < STOOPING.

Caust. *227*.

DRY WITH CONSTANT DESIRE TO SWALLOW.

Sul. *788*.

PAINS IN THROAT 'OUT OF ALL PROPORTION' TO APPARENT CONDITION.

Lach. *493*.

cf Arsenicum – collapse out of proportion.

FISHBONE OR SPLINTER IN THROAT SENSATION.

Arg. nit, Dol. Hepar. Nit. ac Sil. Kali carb. *468*.

TEARING PAINS WHEN COUGHING.

Cistus. *286*.

RAW FEELING.

Aesc. *15*. Ammon. carb. *42*. Arg. nit. *80*, Caust. *227*. Puls. *684*.

CHOKY FEELING.
Ail 27. Chel. 250, Glon. 389.
Ign 430. Lach 493.

< HEAT.
Apis. 74.

STINGING PAINS.
Apis. 74. Caps. 200.

PARCHED.
Cann. 183.

INTENSE THIRST.
Cann. 183. Merc. 542.

DRY WITHOUT THIRST.
Caps. 203.

DIPHTHERITIC.
Ail. 27.

SWOLLEN.
Ail. 28. Bell. (Crot. 332).

SYPHILITIC.
Lac. can. 487.

WITH SCRAPED FEELING.
Med. 531.

BLUE-RED.
Phyt. 652.

SCRAPED SENSATION IN
THROAT WHEN INFLAMMED.
Nux. v. 608.

FAUCES:
dry, very red. Stram. 774.
tickling in . . Bac. (Tub. 834).
with itching throat. Cistus.
286.
inflamed and dry. Cistus. 286.
Sal. ac. 724.
oedema or gangrene of . .
Crot. 336.
ulcers on . . Kali bich. 456,
459, Lach. 498, Sal. ac. 724,

Kali br. 467, Phyt. 652.
white spots. Caps. 203.

FEELS SPASMODICALLY CLOSED.
Caps. 204.

VIOLENT COUGH BEFORE
RISING.
Nux v. 604.

TOUCH OF THROAT CAUSES
GAGGING.
Nux v. 607.

STITCHES CAUSE COUGHING.
Cistus. 286. Lac. can. 490.

FEELING OF LUMP IN.
Lac. can. 487. Lach. 492.

AS IF GRASPED BY THE
THROAT.
Lach. 493.

> SWALLOWING. ONLY TO
RETURN.
Ign. Lac. can. 487.

< TOUCHING THROAT.
Lach. 492. 498.

< FROM SLEEP.
Lach. 492.

< FROM HOT DRINKS.
Lach. 492. Phyt. 652.

SPASM OF GLOTTIS.
Med. 532.

SWOLLEN EXTERNALLY.
Rhus. 712.

AS IF FILLED WITH PLUG.
Ant. crud. 55, Ign. 430- Kali
bich, 459, Psor 676.

SWALLOWING.
painful if 'empty'. Lach. 492.
> swallowing liquids. Lach.
498.

.nroat feels too tight. Lyc. *517*.

results in pain in tonsils.
Merc. *542*.

difficult. Nitric ac. *591*, Phys.
651. Plumbum. *670*, Sal. ac.
724 Stram. *774*. Kali carb. *472*.
Lach. *498* Lac. can. *487, 490*.
must swallow continually.
Caust. *227*.

always trying to swallow.
Cina *284*. Ign. *430*. Lac. can.
487.

almost impossible. Ant. tart.
69, Lach. *497* Hyos. *412*. Lac
can. *490*.

SENSITIVE TO EXTERNAL
TOUCH.
Lach. Lac. can. *487*.

PAINS SHOOT TO EARS WITH
CONSTANT SWALLOWING.
Phyt. Lac. can. *487*. Lach. *497*.

DECOMPOSITION OF MUCOUS
MEMBRANES OF . .
Kreos. *489*.

SPASMS OF PHARYNX.
Iris. *451*.

CANNOT SPEAK LOUDLY.
Ign. *429*.

MUCH HAWKING.
Cistus. *286*.

> FROM EXPECTORATION.
Cistus. *286*.

PARALYSIS.
Caust. *223*. Hyos. *412*.
Plumbum. *670*.

APHONIA.
Caust. *222*. Cina *282*. Collin.
310. Acon. Phos. Spong (Cina
282).

SPUTUM WHITE.
Ant. tart. *64*.

AS IF A STICK IN THE THROAT.
Hepar. Arg. nit. *79. 80*. Arg.
nit. Kali c. Nit. ac. Hepar.
401. 405. Lach. *497*.

< WHEN NOT SWALLOWING.
Cap. *204*. Ign. *430*.

PEPPERMINT TASTE IN MOUTH.
Ver. alb. *854*.

THICK ROPY MUCOUS.
Kali bich. San. *737*.

HOARSENESS > AFTER
TALKING FOR SOME TIME.
Rhus. *710*.

EXPECTORATION. BLOODY.
Crot. Tereb. *810*.

non-viscid thick phlegm. Tub.
833.

PARALYSIS OF ORGANS OF
DEGLUTITION.
Gels. Bapt. *115*. Gels. *382*.

TISSUE ROUND CERVICAL
GLANDS SWOLLEN. CALC.
160.

TINEA KERION
INFLAMMATORY PUSTULES ON
SCALP. see SKIN.

TISSUE SALTS
Silica. Nat. mur. Ferr. phos.
(375.369) Calc. phos. Mag.
phos. Nat. phos. Kali phos.
(Ferr. phos. 377) Mag. phos.
523.

TONGUE

DRY.

Agar. *24*. Ail. *27*, Ars. *98*, Bapt. *113/4*, Bell. *122*. Bry. *145* Calc. *160* Hyos. *412*. Mur. ac. *564*, Nux. mosch. *596*. Pyrogen. *691* Rhus. *708. 712*.

with abdominal tension. Tereb. *811*.

with increase of tympanites. Tereb. *811*.

very dry. Psor. *676*.

BURNING.

Sul. *782*. Tereb. *810*, Caps. *199*. Iris. *450*, Nat. sul. *584*. Sul. *782*.

SWOLLEN.

Merc. *537, 541, 545*. Dulc. *365*. Iod. *433*. Mag. phos. *524*. Crot. *336*. Acon. *9*. Bapt. *113*. Calc. p. (Calc. s. *171*.

BLISTERED.

Graph. *399*. Nat. phos. *577*. Nat. sul. *584*. Lyc. *517*, Med. *531* Nat. mur. *572*.

as if scalded. Ver. vir. *862*, Sang. *730*, Puls. *684*.

PARCHED.

Ail. *27*. Carbo v. *210*.

CRACKED.

Ail. *27*. Calc. fl. (Calc. s. *171*). Kali bich. *453. 455*. Mez. *556*.

MOIST.

Ail. *27*. Merc. *538*. Nat. mur. *576*.

RAW.

Bapt. *113*. Ipec. *441*.

COVERED WITH BURNING VESICLES.

Sal. ac. *724*

FLABBY.

Calc. s. *171*, Camph. *176*. Med. *538*.

PIMPLY.

Calc. p. (Calc. s. *171*).

NUMB.

Borax. *136*. Gels. *385*. Glon. *390*. Nat. mur. *574*.

STIFF.

Borax. *316*. Calc. p. (Calc. s. *171*). Colch. *304*.

COLD.

Camph. *176*. Carbo v. *210, 212*.

TREMBLING.

Camph. *176*.

STICKY.

Carbo v. *210*.

PARALYSED.

Mur. ac. *564*, Opium. *616*. Crot. casc. (Crot *339*) Cup. *345*. Hyos. *412. 415*.

causing stammerings. Caust *224*.

as result of cold. Dulc. *365*.

GANGRENOUS.

Lach. *499*.

ULCERATED.

Bapt. *113, 115*. Kali bich. *455*. Lach. *499*. Lyc. *517*.

PASTY.

Bapt. *114*.

FOUL.

Bapt. *113*. Carbo v. *211*.

FEELS TOO LONG.
Aeth. *19.*

WITH FINE PENETRATING STITCHES.
Acon. *9.*

CRAMPED.
Borax. *136.*

VESICLES ON OR UNDER.
Cham. *239.*

SHOWING IMPRINT OF TEETH.
Chel. *249. 250.* Med. *537/9.*
Merc. *542. 545.*

DIFFICULT TO PROTRUDE.
Lach. Colch. *304, 308.* Lach. *493, 499.*

PROTRUDING.
Crot. *335. 336*

HEAVY – DIFFICULT SPEECH.
Nat. mur. *572.*

BITES TONGUE.
Caust. *224.*

STIFF, AS IF PARALYSED.
Stram. *771.*

SIDES OF TONGUE TURN UP.
Stram. *733.*

CRAMP IN TONGUE.
Ruta *723.*

COVERED WITH VISCID MUCOUS.
Puls. *684.*

LEUKOPLAKIA.
Nitric ac. *588.*

STICKS TO ROOF OF MOUTH.
Nux. mosch. *596. 598/9* San.. *733.*

BITTEN DURING SLEEP.
Theridion. *817.*

SENSATION AS IF TONGUE IS TOO HEAVY.
Ver. alb. *855.*

FEELS TIED UP.
Crot. *336.*

NUMB AFTER A FRIGHT.
Hyos. *415.*

LIKE LEATHER.
Hyos. *414.* San. *733.*

PERFECTLY CLEAN, WITH NAUSEA.
Cina. Ipec. *443.*

CATCHES IN TEETH.
Lach. *497.*

COATED:
creamy or golden-yellow. Nat. phos. *577.*

greenish. Nat. sul. *584.*

dark brown. Rhus. *708.*

dark brown streak down centre. San. *733.*

red streak in centre. Ver. vir. *861.*

white or yellow. Ver vir. *861.*

thick white. *Ant. crud. 52. 56.* Ant. tart. *67,* Bry. *148,* Caust. *227.*

whitish. Ail. *27.* Merc. *541/ 2* Pet. *632.*

milky white. Ant. crud. *53.*

yellow. Ant. crud *53,* Calc. s. *171.* Chel. *247, 250.* Collin. *311* Puls. Kali sul. *475.* Kali bich. *453, 459.*

brown. Ars. *98.* Bapt. *114.*

bluish. Carbo v. *210.*

Colch. *304*. Merc. *545*.
black. Ars. Carbo. v. *211*.
212.

MAPPED.
Tarax. Ran. sc. Rhus. *707*.
Ars. Ran. b. *702* Nat. mur.
571. Rhus. *707*.

with much burning. Ran. sc.
702/3.

SMOOTH, GLOSSY RED.
Crot. Pyrogen. Tereb. *813*.

RED.
Acon. *11*. Ant. tart. *67*. Bapt.
114. Colch. *308*. Ipec. *441* Kali
bich. *453*. *455*, Merc. *545*,
Tereb. *813*.

RED IN MIDDLE.
Caust. *227*.

PAINFUL RED TIP.
Arg. nit. *80*.

WITH RED MARGIN.
Chel. *250*.

RED TIPPED
Crot. *337*. Rhus. *708*.

DARK RED.
Bell. *122*.

RED IN STREAKS.
Ant. tart. *67*. Ars. *98*.

WITH LIVID TIP AND EDGES.
Ail. *27*.

**YELLOW-BROWN STREAK
DOWN CENTRE.**
Bapt. Pyrogen. *691*.

WITH WHITE FUR.
Ail *27*, Calc. p. (Calc. s. *171*)
Pyrogen *691*.

SHINY LIKE A GLASS BOTTLE.
Kali bich. *455, 458*.

INSULAR LARGE PATCHES ON . .
Kali bich. *459*.

CANCER OF . . .
Crot. *336*.

TONSILS

TONSILLITIS.
Caps *200*, Dulc. *363*.

SWOLLEN.
Ammon. carb. *45*, Lac. can.
490 Nitric ac. *591*. Phyt. *654*.

SWOLLEN, BUT NO PAIN.
Bapt. *115*, Cham. *240*.

CHRONIC TONSILLITIS.
Hepar *407*, with hardness of
hearing. Hepar *407*.

**TO HASTEN SUPPURATION, LOW
POTENCIES OF**
Merc. *538*

**TO ABORT SUPPURATION, HIGH
POTENCIES.**
Merc. *538*.

ULCERATED.
Ail. *27*.

WITH SUPPURATION.
Calc. s. *172*. Merc. *542*.

CHRONIC ENLARGEMENT.
Calc. p. *166*.

RED AND SHINING.
Lac. can. *490*.

RED.
Nitric ac. *591*.

WITH YELLOW STREAK.
Nitric ac. *591*.

WITH PAIN ALTERNATING FROM
SIDE TO SIDE.
Lac. can. *489.*

BURNING, SMARTING PAIN.
Caps. *200.*

WITH SMALL ULCERS.
Nitric ac. *591.*

WITH DEEP ULCERS.
Ail. *28.*

TORTICOLLIS
WRY-NECK. see NECK.

TOTALITY OF SYMPTOMS.
Stram. *780.*

TRACHITIS
INFLAMMATION OF THE
TRACHEA.
Ant. tart. *68.*

TRACHOMA
Apis. *75.* see EYES.

TRISMUS
LOCKJAW. see FACE.

TUBERCULAR DIATHESIS
Agar. *21. 22.* Calc. *155.* Dros.
352. Theridion. *817* Nat. sul.
585.

WITH EMACIATION.
Brom. *140,* Sil. *758.*

CONSUMPTION.
Calc. *162.*

FEVER.
Calc. *163.*

RESISTANCE TO TUBERCLE
RAISED.
Dros. *353.*

TUBERCULAR SINUSES.
Tub. Sil. Dros. *357.*

TUBERCULAR ABDOMEN.
Sul. Lil. tig. Tub. bov. Dros.
358.

TYMPANITES
DISTENSION OF THE ABDOMEN
DUE TO GAS OR AIR IN THE
INTESTINES OR PERITONEAL
CAVITY. see ABDOMEN.

TYPHLITIS
INFLAMMATION OF CAECUM.
Plumbum. *670.*

TYPHOID
Bapt. *115.* Bell. *120,* Calc. *163.*
Carbo v. *213.* Phos. ac. *639*
Nux mosch. *599.* Colch. *304.*
Crot. *338.* (trachitis) Mur.ac.
565 Pyrogen. *812.*

TYPHUS
Arn. *90,* Bapt. *114.* Hyos. *408.*
Mur. ac. *564.* Phos. *647.*
Tereb. *812.* Bry, alternating
with Rhus. *707.*

U

ULCERS
BURNING.
Ars. Tarent. *809,* Ars. *94. 98.*
Carbo. v. *213.* Kreos. *482.*
at night. Carbo v. *211. 213*

INDURATED.
Calc. *157*. Kreos. *480*.
malignant. Calc. *157*. Cistus.
287. Kreos. *480 482*.

VARICOSE.
Carbo v. *210*. Caust. *230*.
Pyrogen. *696*

FISTULOUS.
Caust. *230*.

GANGRENOUS.
Cistus. *288*, Kreos. *482*.

DUODENAL.
Graph. 398, Med. *530*.
Ornithogalum. *620/1*.

GASTRIC.
Crot. *398*. *Graph. 398*.
Ornithogalum. (Graph. *398*)

GASTRIC, WITH HAEMOPTYSIS.
Ornithogalum. *620/1*

BLEEDING.
Hepar. *405*. Merc. *544*, Mez.
555.

SYPHILITIC.
Pet. *631*.

VERY RED.
Lac. can. *490*.

DARK GLISTENING.
Lac. can. *490*.

YELLOW.
Kali bich. *459*.

PURPLE.
Aesc. *15*. Carbo v. *213*.

DARK, PUTRID.
Bapt. *115*.

WITH BLACKISH PATCHES.
Carbo v. *210*, Con. *330*.

WITH THICK WHITISH-YELLOW
SCABS.
Mez. *552*.

VESICLES ROUND ULCERS.
Mez. *552*.

WITH LARDACEOUS BASE.
Merc. *537*.

SENSATION OF COLDNESS IN . .
Merc. *538*. Sil. *756*.

WITHOUT ANY SENSATIONS.
Opium. *615*.

ROUND, AS IF PUNCHED OUT.
Kali bich. *453. 459, 461*. Kali
bich. Phyt. *652*.

> FROM COLD.
Ledum. *504*.

TO HELP DISCHARGE AND
HEALING.
Hepar *403*.

VERY SENSITIVE. CANNOT BEAR
TOUCH.
Lach. Hepar *402*, Mez. *555*.

DEEP IN TONSILS.
Ail. *28*. Kali bich. *456*.

INTERNAL.
Arg. nit. *78/9*.

PERIOSTEAL.
Asaf. *103/4*.

OF MOUTH.
Bapt. *115*, Borax. *133*, Iod.
433.

APHTHAE OF CHILDREN.
Borax. *132*, Bry. Borax. *133/5*.
of nipples. Borax. *132*.
of stomach. Borax. *134*.

PHAGADENIC ON JOINTS OF
FINGERS AND TOES.
Borax. *137.*

OF STOMACH (GASTRIC).
Crot. *338, Graph. 398.*
Ornithogalum (Graph *398*)
Kreos *480*, Kali bich. *460.*
Mez. *553.*

CHRONIC STOMACH ULCERS.
Brom. *141.*

SUBCUTANEOUS.
Puls. Ran. b. *702* Ran., sc. *702.*

OLD LEG ULCERS.
Kali bich. *455.*

OLD DEEP ULCERS ON ANKLE
AND SHIN.
Cistus. *288.* Kali bich. *455.*

OLD PUTRID ULCERS
SPREADING.
Chel. *251.* Kreos. *482.* Ars.
Dulc. *364.*

ON WRIST.
Kali bich. *461.*

ON LUNGS.
Kali carb. *473.*

OF SOFT PALATE.
Hepar. *404.*

OF LEGS.
Sil. *754.*

ABOUT THE NAILS.
Sil. *754.*

OF MUCOUS MEMBRANES. OF
STOMACH AND BOWELS.
Sal. ac. *724.*

OF FACE AND LIPS.
Con. *328.*

WITH:
feeble relaxed tissues. Carbo
v. *210.*

stagnating capillaries. Carbo
v. *210.*

infiltration of mucous
membranes. Brom. *140.*

vomiting of blood
(Haematemesis).
Arg. nit. *79.* Kreos *482.*

VERY SENSITIVE.
Asaf. *103. 104.*

URAEMIA
CONDITION RESULTING FROM
RETENTION OF POISONS. see
URINE.

URINE
BURNING.
Merc. *539.* Nat. sul. *585.* Ran.
b. *699* Canth. Cann. Tereb.
813 Allium. *32.* Borax *135.*
Lyc. (Calc. *153*) Cann. *183.*
Canth. *193.*

during micturition. Tereb.
814. Camph. *176.* Cann. *183,*
Canth. 195/6 Colch. *309.* Caps.
204. Staph. *763.* Ran. b. *699.*

before micturition. Cann. *183.*
Canth. *198.*

after micturition. Cann. *183,*
Canth. *198.* Caps. *201.*

when NOT micturating.
Staph. 766.

STINGING PAINS BEFORE
MICTURITION.
Cann. *183.*

during and after micturition.
Cann. *183*.

CUTTING PAINS IN URETHA
BEFORE, DURING AND AFTER
URINATION.
Canth. 193. 195/6 198.

DIFFICULT MICTURITION.
Plumbum. *668*.

POLYURIA (PROFUSE).
Merc. *543*. Mur. ac. *563, 565*,
Vib. *866*. Nat. phos. *576* Nat
sul. *585*. Phos. ac. *563*. Tarent.
801. San. *736*. Allium. *32*.
Cann. *183*. Caust. *228*. Kreos.
479.

PROFUSE FROM 6–7 P.M.
Bry. *146*.

PROFUSE WITH WEAKNESS.
Calc. p. *168*.

> AFTER EMISSION OF PROFUSE
WATERY URINE.
Gels. *385/6* Ign. *425*.

SCANTY.
Apis. *72*. Canth. *193*. Crot.
337. Cup. *344*. Iris. *452*. Med.
535 Nitric ac. *591*, Puls. *684*.
Vib. *866*. San. *734*. Thuja. *819*.

FREQUENT ATTEMPTS TO
URINATE.
Arn. *89*. Caps. *201*. Staph. *763*.
Kreos. *479* Colch. *309*. Cicuta.
263. Nux v. *607*.

ANXIOUS DESIRE TO URINATE.
San. *734*. Staph. *763*. Arn. *89*.
Canth. *193*. *198* Caust. *228*.
Ign. *431*. Coloc. *319*.
if cold. Dulc. *365*.

SUPPRESSED.
Stram. *775*. Apis. *72*. Arum.
triph. Ail. *29*. Bell. *122*. Canth.
195

RETENTION.
with a full bladder. Opium.
614. 616.

spasmodic. Tereb. *812*.

except when standing. Caust.
224. (Dribbles while sitting.
Sarsaparilla (Caust. *224*).

URGING DUE TO IMPENDING
FEVER.
Pyrogen. *691*.

FEELING SOME URINE STILL IN
BLADDER.
Hepar *405*. Kali bich. *460*.

URGING TO URINATE.
Ferr. *372*. Kreos. *479*. Lil. tig.
509. 512. Nux v. *607* Lyc. *518*.
Nat. phos. *578*. Phos. ac. *638*
(with scanty discharge).

OBLIGED TO WAIT FOR URINE
TO PASS.
Hepar. *405*.

CANNOT PASS WITHOUT
STRAINING.
Alum. *36*. Lil. tig. *509*. Mur.
ac. *564*.

HAS TO WAIT A LONG TIME FOR
URINE TO PASS.
Arn. *89*. Bell. *125*. Lyc. *515*.

CAN ONLY URINATE LYING
DOWN.
Kreos. *483*.

CAN ONLY URINATE WHEN
PASSING STOOL.
Mur. ac. *563*.

URINATES WHEN PASSING
STOOL.
Alum. *36*.

PAINS IN NECK OF BLADDER
WHILE URINATING.
Nux. v. *607*.

INEFFECTUAL URGING TO
URINATE.
Bell. *125*, Nux v. *607*. Opium.
614.

INVOLUNTARY:
during first sleep. Sepia. *741*.
when passing wind. Mur. ac.
563.
when walking, coughing,
sneezing. Nat. mur. *573*.
in drops. Arn. *89*.
< motion. Bry. *143*. Ferr. *370*.
on hearing running water.
Hydrophobinum. (Hyos. *412*).
at night. Caust. *228*, Ferr. *370*,
Sepia. *741*.
due to paralysis of sphincter.
Caust. *224*.

DRIBBLING.
Cann. *183*. *188*, Caust. *227*.

DRIBBLES WHEN SITTING AND
WALKING.
Puls. *684*.

CRIES AND SCREAMS BEFORE
URINATION.
Borax. *135*.

< BEFORE URINATION.
Borax. *135*.

AT EVERY COUGH.
Caust. *224*.

WITH TICKLING IN URETHA.
Ferr. *372*.

ITCHING ORIFICE OF URETHA.
Caust. *228*, Nux. v. *607*.

WITH DIARRHOEIA.
Alum. *36*, Sal. ac. *725*.

TENESMUS OF NECK OF
BLADDER.
Arn. *89*. Canth. *193*. *194*. *198*.

OFFENSIVE.
Sal. ac. *725*.

FETID.
Bapt. *115*.

PUNGENT AMMONIACAL SMELL.
Asaf. *102*.

VERY ACID.
Arn. *89*.

GELATINOUS.
Crot. *333*. *337*

TURBID.
Dulc. *364*. Graph. *399*. Nat.
mur. *569*.

ALBUMINOUS.
Gels. *383*. Glon. *393*.
Plumbum. *667*. Tereb. *810/1*.

CLOUDY WITH SEDIMENT.
Ipec. *445*, Tereb. *812*.

SMELLS OF VIOLETS.
Tereb. *810*, *812*.

CLOUDY AND SMOKY.
Tereb. *810*, *813/4*.

HAEMATURIA.
Tereb. *812*, Canth. *194*. *198*.
Ledum. *504*. Tereb. *811*.

WATERY.
Ign. Thuja. *819*. Cocc. *296*.
Sepia. *742*.

ALKALINE AND ROPY.
Kali bich. *460*.

WITH RED SAND.
Lyc. *515. 518.*

WITH RED FLAKES.
Mez. *555.* Sepia. *742.*

MILKY.
Lyc. *518.*

STRONG SMELLING.
Med. *532.* Nitric ac. *588. 591.*

HIGHLY COLOURED.
Med. *535.*

COLD.
Nitric. ac. (Con. *330*).

LIKE INK.
Colch. *307.* Crot. *333.*

PALE.
Colch. *305.*

VERY YELLOW OR DARK
BROWN.
Chel. *247. 251.*

BROWN.
Arn. *89.*

WITH SANDY DEPOSITS.
Lyc. Ledum *504.*

FEELS COLD AS IT PASSES.
Agar. Nitric ac. *588.*

THICK WITH PUS.
Arn. *89.*

URAEMIA.
Ammon. carb. *44.* Plumbum.
665. Tereb. *811.* Urtica. *848.*

URAEMIC COMA.
Plumbum. *665.*

FORKED STREAM.
Thuja. *828.*

INFLAMES SKIN.
Lyc. *515.*

WITH SMARTING AND BURNING
IN PUDENDA.
Kreos. *479.*

ITCHING FROM CONTACT.
Merc. *539.*

INCONTINENCE IN CHILDREN.
Nat. phos. *576.*

ITCHING DURING MICTURITION.
Pet. *632.*

INTERMITS.
Con. *323/4 327.*

UTERUS

BURNING IN . .
Tereb. *812.*

CRAMP IN . .
Vib. *866.*

BRUISED.
Arn. Bellis. *131.*

CONGESTED.
Caul. *216.*

GRIPING AND PINCHING IN . .
Cham. *2 40*

HAEMORRHAGES.·
Vib. *866.* Bell. *122.* Caul. *219.*
220. Ipec. *441. 443. 446* Lac.
can. *488.* Pyrogen. *694.*
bright and stringy. Lac. can.
488.
dark and stringy. Croc. (Lac.
can. *488*).
in gushes. *Ipec. 448.*

SPASMODIC PAINS IN . .
Cimic (Actea racemosa) *271/2.*
Mag. mur. (Caul. *217*) Secale.
(Caul. *218*) Gels. *386.*

210

SEVERE NEURALGIC PAINS IN . .
Lil. tig. *512*.

LABOUR-LIKE PAINS IN . .
Opium. *613*. Vib. *865*.

PAINS < TOUCH OR JAR.
Lil. tig. *512*.

UTERINE BEARING DOWN:
as if uterus would come out.
Plat. Pall. *625* Sepia *743*.

with haughtiness,
overbearing. Plat. Pall. *625*.

with dull indifference. Sepia.
(Pall. *625*).

with aimless worries. Lil. tig.
(Pall. *625*).

> holding breath and bearing
down. Pyrogen. *691. 693*.

PAINFUL VULVA.
Plat. *662*.

PROLAPSUS.
Caul. *219*, Cimic. *277* (if
symptoms agree) Sepia *742*.
Plat. *662*.

with hunger, constipation,
dragging down feeling. *Sepia
747*.

with diarrhoea. Pod. Collin.
313. Ferr. *373*.

with piles. Collin. *313*.

CANCER OF . .
Iod. *435*. Kreos *478*. Merc.
540.

with profuse haemorrhages.
Iod. *435*.

MIOMA (TUMOURS) UTERI.
Calc. s. *172*.

FIBROID TUMOURS.
Con. *323*.

ULCERS ON NECK OF . .
Kreos. *479*.

POLYPS.
Calc. p. *167. 168*.

HYPERTROPHY.
Helonias. Fraxinus, Bellis.
131.

as if everything would fall out.
Bell. *122*.

DISPLACEMENT.
Calc. p. *166*, Lil tig. *509*.

CONTRACTIONS, FEEBLE.
Caul. *219*.

SUB INVOLUTION.
Caul. *219*.

UTERINE EPILEPSY AND
HYSTERIA.
Cimic. *274*.

> AFTER FLOW FROM . .
Cimic. *277*.

FEELS CONSTRICTED.
Cactus. (Gels. *384*).

WITH NAUSEA.
Ipec. *443*.

EXCESSIVE ITCHING IN UTERUS.
Plat. *662*.

TO HELP EXPEL CONTENTS.
Pyrogen. *695*.

MUST SUPPORT PARTS BY
HAND.
San. *732*.

MUST SIT DOWN TO STOP HER
INSIDES COMING OUT.
Lil. tig. Sepia *738. 747*.

PRESSURE IN UTERUS, AS IF
EVERYTHING WOULD ISSUE
THROUGH VULVA.
Sepia. *741/2, 747.*

HYSTERICAL CONVULSIONS
FROM UTERINE IRRITATION.
Vib. *865.*

ABORTIFACIENT AND ECHOLIC.
Cimic. *274.*

V

VACCINATION
EFFECTS OF . .
Thuja, Sil. Ant. tart. *70.*
Thuja. *823/5.*

AILMENTS RESULTING FROM . .
Sil. *756. Thuja 820/1.*

ANTIDOTE IN EARLY STAGES.
Thuja. *822.*

VACCINOSIS
AILMENTS RESULTING FROM
VACCINATION.
Cean. *233.* Thuja *821. 823/5.*
Tub. *841.*

VAGINISM
A SPASMODIC CONTRACTION OF
THE VAGINA.
Plumbum. *668.*

VAGUS NERVE
Cocc. *291.*

VARICOCELE
VEINS OF TESTICLES
DISTENDED. see
GENITALIA.

VARIOLA
SMALL POX.
Ant. tart. *69,* Cup. *348.*

VEINS and ARTERIES
BURNING.
Ars. *94.* Calc. *164.* Carbo v.
207.

VARICES BURN LIKE FIRE.
Ars. *97.*

FEELING OF BLOOD BOILING.
Aur. *110.*

AS IF COLD WATER RAN
THROUGH.
Ver. alb. *856.*

PURPLE.
Aesc. *12. 15.*

CONGESTION OF . .
Aesc. *12.*

VARICOSE VEINS.
Carbo v. *207, 210.* Puls. Ferr.
367.

possibly caused by spleen
enlargement. Cean. *234.*

discomfort of . . Bell. *130.*
Calc. *157.*

ENLARGED, PUFFY.
Brom. *141.* Carbo v. *207.* Chel.
251. Glon. *391* Lach. *493.*
Amyl. nit. (Glon. *391*).

VENOUS TURGESSENCE.
Carbo v. *207.*

VENOUS STAGNATION.
Thuja. Carbo v. *210.*

HYPERAEMIA.
Ferr. phos. 378.

ANEURISM.
Lyc. *522,* Ran. sc. (Ran. b. *703*).

LAZY, RELAXED.
Carbo v. *207.*

PARALYSED.
Carbo v. *207.*

PAINS IN JUGULAR AND CAROTID.
Crot. casc. (Crot. *340*).

VENEREAL DISEASES.
Merc. *540.*

VERMIFUGES
see CONVULSIONS.

VERTIGO
SEASICKNESS.
Theridion. *815.* Con. *331.*

< RIDING IN CARRIAGE OR BOAT.
Cocc. 293/5 Con. *322.* Pet. *629.*

FROM DOWNWARD MOTION.
Borax. *132. 135/6* Ferr. *370.* Con. *329.*

WITH:
sleepiness. Aeth. *20.*
Nausea. Ail. *27.* Calc. *159.* Colch. *295/6* Theridion. *815.*
vomiting. Ail. *27,* Calc. *159.* Chel. *249. Cocc. 291.*
eyes out of focus. Alum. *40.*

sensation of falling. Calc. *159.*
headache. Calc. *159*
pain in liver. Chel. *249.*
confusion. Cocc. *296.*
eyes open. Con. *331.*
dimness of vision. Cycl. *350.*
momentary loss of consciousness. Nux. v. *603.*

VIOLENT.
Ars. *93.* Cann. *182/3.*

'VISUAL'.
Alum. *40,* Gels. *385.*

SUDDEN.
Cimic. *276.*

PERSISTENT, AFTER EPILEPTIC ATTACKS.
Viscum. *867.*

DURING EPILEPTIC SPASMS.
Calc. *159.*

ON:
rising from chair. Bry. *148. 150* Cocc. *296.* Ferr. *370.*
turning head. Calc. *155. 159.* Con. *322. 324. 327.*
seeing running water. Ferr. *371.*
walking over water, on a bridge. Ferr. *370.*
shutting eyes. Lach. Thuja. *Theridion. 815/8* Arn. *88,* Chel. *249.*
opening eyes. Tabacum. (Theridion. *818*).
looking UPwards. Puls. Sil. (Theridion. *818*) Phos. (Con. *325*).

seeing moving objects (from paresis of accommodation) Cocc. *295* Con. *322*.

DURING A MEAL.
Ammon. carb. *42*.

ON HIGH PLACES.
Calc. *159*.

IN ADDISON'S DISEASE.
Calc. *159*.

OBJECTS SEEM TO MOVE IN A CIRCLE.
Cicuta. *264*, Con. *322. 325*.

FROM CONGESTION TO PARTS OF BRAIN OR HEAD.
Ferr. phos. *379*, Iod. *433*.

INCLINED TO FALL TO LEFT.
Sal. ac. *724*.

GIDDINESS IN HORIZONTAL POSITION.
Sal. ac. *724*.

DARE NOT MOVE HER EYES,
Plat. *662*.

IN MORNING, WITH FALLING WHEN STANDING.
Phos ac. *637*.

IN EVENING WHEN STANDING, WALKING.
Phos. ac. *637*.

AS IF FLOATING IN AIR.
Lac. can. *490*.

AS IF DRUNK.
Ferr. *371*. Puls. *683*. Cocc. *296*. Pet. *629*.

< MOTION.
Bry. *143*, Paeonia. *622*, Phos. *645*.

< LYING DOWN.
Con. *322. 325*. Phos. (Con. *325*) Rhod. *705*.

ONLY ON LEFT SIDE.
Iod. *433*.

< ON WAKING.
Lach. *497/8*. Lyc. *516* Nitric ac. *590*, Pet. *629*.

< ON WAKING AND SEEING OBJECTS 'TRANSPARENTLY'
Cyclamen. (Con. *325*).

< ON CLOSING EYES.
Lach. *498*.

< WHEN SITTING.
Puls. *683*.

< IN THE OPEN AIR.
Phos. (Con. *325*).

< AFTER EATING.
Phos. (Con. *325*).

< IN THE EVENING.
Phos. (Con. *325*).

< ON TURNING OVER ON TO RIGHT SIDE.
Cean. (Con. *325*).

VETERINARY

VIOLENT COUGH IN SHEEP.
Dros. *353/4*.

WASTING AWAY IN SHEEP.
Dros. *353/4*.

(PROLONGED USE OF DROSERA INDUCES TUBERCULIZATION.
Dros. *254* and *therefore use of potentised Drosera cures it.*)

SWELLING OF CERVICAL AND OTHER GLANDS IN CATS.
Dros. *354*.

SOWS EAT THEIR YOUNG.
Ferr. phos. *379.*

ANTHRAX.
Kreos. *482.*

LAME HORSES.
Ledum. *502.*

PUNCTURED WOUNDS, NAILS
ETC.
Ledum *503.*

METEORISM (BLOATING) IN
COWS.
Colch. Mag. phos. *525. 527.*

ACTINOMYOCOSIS IN CATTLE
(WOODY TONGUE).
Nitric ac. *589.*

COAGULATED MILK.
Phty. *650.*

LUMPS IN COW'S BAGS.
Phyt. *650.*

SWOLLEN UDDERS.
Phyt. *650.*

STRINGY MILK.
Phyt. *651.*

RETAINED PLACENTA.
Pyrogen. *696.*

INDIFFERENCE TO OFFSPRING.
Sepia. *744.*

EPILEPSY IN HORSES.
Viscum. *867.*

VITAL FORCE
VITAL POWERS DIMINISHED.
Carbo v. *209, 213,* Crot. *336,*
Opium. *616.*

ADYNAMIC (GREAT DEPRESSION
OF VITAL POWER) FEVER.
Carbo v. *213.*

LACK OF VITAL REACTION.
Psor. *672.*

VITAMINS
Ferr. phos. *376.* Calc. p. *170.*

VOMITING
VIOLENT.
Acon. *10.* Aeth. *17. 19.* Ail.
26/7 Ant. crud. *55.* Med. *534.*
Con. *328.* Colch. *302. 307.* Ver.
alb. *854.*

EXCESSIVE, CONTINUOUS.
Ver. alb. *854.*

CONSTANT.
Ars. *93. 99,* Ipec. *441.*
Plumbum. *668.*

WITHOUT RELIEF.
Ars. *99.*

DESIRE TO, WITH SENSATION AS
IF HEAD WERE IN A VICE.
Arg. nit. *80.* Caps. *203.*

CONSTANT RETCHING.
Crot. *333.*

DIFFICULT TO VOMIT.
Ant. tart. *65,* Cham. *240.*

UNTIL HE BECOMES FAINT.
Ant. tart. *69.*

SIMULTANEOUS VOMITING AND
PURGING.
Ars. Arg. nit. *79.*

AFTER FOOD.
Ars. *94.* Brom. *141.* Ferr. *370.*

DUE TO SPLEEN ENLARGEMENT.
see Cean *234.*

DURING MEASLES.
Ant. crud. *54.*

215

DISPOSITION TO, AFTER
EATING.
Ant. crud. *52.*

HUNGRY AFTERWARDS.
Aeth. *19.*

IN CHILDREN.
Aeth. *18.* Camph. *173.* xv, Ars.
99.

AFTER SOUR WINE.
Ant. crud. *53.*

DESIRE TO . .
Ant. crud. *53.*

AFTER MIDNIGHT.
Ferr. *370.*

ONLY AFTER EATING.
Ferr. *372.* Sepia. (Ferr. *373*).

FROM WARM FOOD, WATER,
ROOM.
Phos. *644.*

VOMITS WATER WHEN IT
BECOMES WARM IN STOMACH.
Phos. Pyrogen. *690.*

PERIODICAL.
Iris. *451.*

REGULARLY EVERY MORNING
AND EVENING.
Psor. *677.*

CADAVEROUS SMELLING.
Kreos. *478.*

'SYMPATHETIC' E.G. OF
PHTHISIS, CANCER, KIDNEY
DISEASE.
Kreos. *481.*

INCLINATION TO . .
Nux v. *605.* Puls. *684.*

AFTER CHLOROFORM.
Phos. *644.*

AT SIGHT OF WATER DURING
PREGNANCY.
Phos. *644.*

WITHOUT NAUSEA.
Med. *531.*

< FROM . . .
Ferr. *371.*

< LYING ON RIGHT SIDE OR
BACK.
Crot. *336. 338.*

< ACIDS, OYSTERS, TOBACCO
SMOKE.
Brom. *141.*

< WARM THINGS, HOT DRINKS.
Brom. *141.*

< MOTION.
Bry. *143.* Cocc. *291. 296.*
Colch. *308.*

< COLD WATER.
San. *734.*

WITH:
exhaustion. Ammon. carb. *45.*
diarrhoeia. Ant. crud. *55,* Arg.
nit. *80.* Ars. *96.* Kreos. *480.*
prostration. Ant. tart. *62.*
cold sweat. Camph. *176.*
burning in epigastrium.
Colch. *307.*
cold feeling in epigastrium.
Kreos. *480.*
collapse, very slow pulse. Ver.
vir. *861.*
headache. Sang. *729.*
eructations of food. Phos.
Ferr. *373.*
flatulence from acid stomach.
Nux. mosch. *596.*

216

OF:

sour curds. Aeth. *18*, Kreos. *479*. Nat. phos. *576*. San. *734*. Iris. *450/1*.

blood. Carbo v. *211*. Crot. *336*. Ferr. phos. *380*.

bilious matter. Chel. *247*.

pregnancy. Chel. *250*. Nux. mosch. *596*.

cerebral rather than bilious origin. Cocc. *291*.

migraine. Cocc. *291*.

cerebral tumours. Cocc. *291*.

seasickness. Cocc. *296*, Con. *331*. Kreos. *480*. San. *734*. Caps. *200. 202*.

bile. Crot. *335. 338*. Iris. *451*. Nat. sul. *584*.

ropy mucous. Iris. *450*.

drunkards. Kali bich. *453. 458. 460*.

sour fluid. Nat phos. *575*. Nux. v. *605*.

VULNERARIES
ANYTHING USED IN HEALING WOUNDS
Bellis. *127/8*.

W

WALKING
INABILITY TO WITH EYES SHUT.
Alum. *37*.

BACKWARD IN LEARNING.
Calc. *163*, Caust. *229*.

LOSS OF POWER IN LIMBS ON WALKING.
Calc. *163*.

unable to go upstairs.
Calc. *163*.

STOOPING AND BENDING FORWARD.
Sul. *791*.

WARTS
Ammon carb. *42*. *Thuja*, Dulc. *Caust. 224*. Nat. sul. *582*.

ON HANDS.
Ant. crud. *58*.

ON HANDS AND FACE.
Caust. *225*, Dulc. *365*.

LARGE PEDUNCULATED.
Caust. *230*. Nitric ac. *593*.

LARGE, FLESHY, SMOOTH OR FLAT.
Dulc. *364/5*.

BLEEDING READILY.
Nitric ac. *593*.

SOFT AND MOIST.
Nitric ac. *593*.

STICKING AND PRICKING.
Nitric ac. *593*.

ON FACE AND LEGS.
Kali br. *466*.

ABOUT ANUS AND GENITALS.
Thuja, Nat. sul. *582*.

WEAKNESS
AFTER FLU.
Abrot. *2*.

UNABLE TO HOLD HEAD UP.
Abrot. Aeth. *18*.

EXHAUSTED.
Aeth. *19*. Colch. *308*, Nat.
mur. *573*.

MIND AND BODY WEAK.
Ammon. carb. *41*. *44*. Lach.
498.

WITHOUT APPARENT CAUSE.
Ammon. carb. *41*. *44*. Nitric
ac. *593*.

OF ALL SENSES.
Anac. *48*.

**OUT OF ALL PROPORTION TO
OTHER SYMPTOMS.**
Ars. *97*.

JUST TIRED AND BELOW PAR.
China. *257*.

FROM LOSS OF SLEEP.
Cocc. (China. *257*) Cocc. *293*.

**FROM OVER-EXERTION,
MUSCULAR FATIGUE.**
Arn. (China. *257*).

GREAT SENSE OF WEAKNESS.
Cocc. *293*, Nat. mur. *573*.
Phos. *647*. Ver. alb. *855*.

OF WHOLE BODY, ON RISING.
Lach. *498*.

EASILY TIRED.
Nat. mur. *573*.

WITH TREMBLING LIMBS.
Nitric ac. *593*.

WEATHER
> COLD.
Ledum. (Colch. *306*) Picric ac.
657.

< COLD.
Colch. *306*. Kreos. *483*. Nat.
mur. *570*. Phos. *644*. *Phyt. 651*

Psor. *678*. Ran. b. *701*, Rhus.
Rhod. *704*.

< COLD ROUND HEAD.
Baryta carb. Sil. *756*.

< COLD WET.
Rhod. *705*. *Dulc. 363*, Rhus.
Ammon carb *43*. Acon. *5*.
Puls. *682* Sil. (Hepar *401*) Nux
mosch. *599*. *Bellis. 128*.

**< COLD BATHING OR FALLING
INTO WATER.**
Bellis, Ant. crud. *57*.

< COLD DAMP.
Ant. crud. *58*, Dulc. (Bry. *147*)
Colch. *303*. Phyt. *651*.

< COLD DRY.
Hepar. *407*. Nux. v. Apis. *72*.
Calc. p. *167* Acon. *5*.

< COLD DRY EAST WIND.
Acon. Asaf. Caust. Hepar.
Kali c. Nux. v. Sep. Spong.
(Bry. *147*) Caust. *222*.

> COLD AIR.
Puls. Aesc. *16*. Puls. Arg. nit.
78. Camph. *176*. Nux. mosch.
599 Puls. Kali sul. *475*.

> WARM AIR.
Caust. *226*. Colch. *306*. Sil.
(Hepar *401*) Kreos. *483*. Phos.
644.

< HEAT.
Ant. crud. *57*. *58*. Apis. *72*.
Arg. nit. *78*. *82*. Nat. mur. *570*
Kali bich. *459*.

< OPEN AIR.
Allium. *30*. Kreos. *483*. Nux.
mosch. *599*.

> DAMP WET WEATHER.
Sang. *729*. Caust. *226*. Lach.
496. Med. *532*.

< WET WARM WEATHER.
Lach. Carbo v. Sil. *Nat. sul.
580,* Tub. *837*. Hepar. *401*.

< DRY.
Nux. v. 601.

< WET.
Picric ac. *657*. Rhus. Rhod.
704.

> OPEN AIR.
Puls. Lyc. *519*. Plat. *659*. *Puls.
681*. Rhus. *711*.

MENTAL SYMPTOMS. > OPEN
AIR.
Cann. *180.*

< MILD.
Lach. *496.*

CHANGE OF WEATHER.
Psor. *678*. Baryta carb. Sil.
756. Tub. *837* Calc. *159*, Nux.
mosch. *599*. Rhod. Phos. Pet.
632. Rhod. *704.*

< CHANGE OF WEATHER FROM
WARM TO COLD.
Dulc. *365.*

< SEA AIR.
Nat. sul. *585.*

< GETTING WET.
Rhus. *715.*

< SUDDEN CHILL FROM WET
COLD WHEN ONE IS HOT.
Bellis *128/9* Dulc. (Bry. *147*).

> IN SUNSHINE. Plat. *659*. < IN
SUNSHINE. Nat. mur. (Plat.
659).

< WIND.
Nitric ac. *586*. Nux. mosch.
599. Nux v. 601.

< CLOUDY.
Lach. 496.

< ANY ELECTRIC CHANGES.
Rhod. *705*. Tub. *837.*

< THUNDERSTORMS.
Tub. *837*. Sepia. Phos. *641*.
Nat. c. Phos. Psor. Rhod. Pet.
632. 629 Nat. phos. *577*. Nitric
ac. *586*. *Rhod. 704*. Psor. *678.*
Rhod. (Caul. *220*).

< Spring.
Lach. *496.*

< IN HEATED ROOMS.
Puls. Kali sul. *475*. Puls. *681.
686.*

< EXTERNAL WARMTH.
Puls. *685.*

WHITLOWS
ACUTE INFLAMMATIONS OF
DEEP-SEATED TISSUES OF
THE FINGERS.
Bell. *127.*

WHOOPING COUGH
Arn. *89*. Chel. *249*. Cina. *282*.
Dros. *352*. Viscum. *868.*

EPIDEMIC.
Dros. (Ver. alb. *850*) (*30* C one
dose only) Dros. *354*, Kali
carb. (Dros. *356*).

VIOLENT.
Cup. *343*. Ferr. *371.*

ALLEVIATION AND ANTIDOTING
EFFECTS OF DROSERA.
Camph. (Dros. *355*).

AFTER DROSERA HAS
RELIEVED SEVERE
SYMPTOMS.
Cina *282*.

WITH TEARING PAIN IN THE
LARYNX.
Allium. *31*.

WITH INDIGESTION, VOMITING
AND FLATULENCE.
Allium *31*.

WITH VIOLENT SPASMODIC
BREATHING.
Cup. *343*. *346*. Ledum. *507*.

> COLD WATER.
Cup. *343*.

WITH VOMITING.
Ferr. *371*. Ipec. *446*.

WITH NOSEBLEED.
Ipec. *446*.

WITH STRINGY MUCOUS.
Kali bich. *460*.

WITH BAGLIKE SWELLING
BETWEEN UPPER LID AND
BROW.
Kali carb. *471*.

< 3 A.M.
Kali carb. *471*.

SEVERE COUGH AFTER . . .
Sang. *729*.

FACE LIVID OR BLUE.
Cup. *343*.

FINGER NAILS DISCOLOURED
Cup *343*.

EYES TURNED UP.
Cup. *343*.

WORMS
IN CHILDREN.
Abrot. *2*. Calc. *157*.

TAPEWORMS.
Calc. *161*. Graph. (Calc. *161*)
Cina *279, 280* Plat *660*.

ASCARIDES.
Calc. *161*. Cina. *280*.

LUMBRICI — ROUND WORMS.
Nat. phos. (Cina *278*) Cina.
280. Nat. phos. *575*.

THREADWORMS.
Cina *279*, Ferr. *370*, Nat. phos.
576.

HELMINTHIASIS.
Cina. *280/1*.

RINGWORM.
Dulc. *364*.

PINWORMS.
Med. *535*.

CAUSING IRRITATION LEADING
TO SQUINTING.
Nat. phos. *576*.

KILLED BY ONIONS.
Allium. *32*.

WORRY (anxiety)
ABOUT TRIFLES.
Acon. *5*. *8*. Mur. ac. *564*.

GENERAL ANXIETY.
Ail. *26/8*. Ammon. carb. *41*.
Ars. *98*. Platt. *661*.

MAKES HIM WALK RAPIDLY.
Arg. nit. *79*.

FAINT, ANXIOUS.
Ars. *100*.

OVERANXIOUS.
Borax. *134*.

TALKS ABOUT BUSINESS.
Bry. *147.*

WITH RESTLESSNESS.
Calc. *158.* Camph. *176.* Iod. *435/6.* Mur. ac. *564.* Plat. *661.*

< TOWARDS EVENING.
Calc. *158.* Camph. *174.* Carbo v. *212.*

PRECORDIAL ANXIETY.
Camph. *174.*

< LYING DOWN.
Carbo v. *212.*

< AWAKENING.
Carbo v. *212.*

< CLOSING EYES.
Carbo v. *212.*

EXCESSIVE WORRY.
Caust. *226.* Ver. alb. *855.*

AFFECTED BY SAD STORIES.
Cicuta. *262.*

SUDDEN EXTREME ANXIETY.
Cocc. *296.*

ANXIETY AS AFTER COMMITTING A CRIME.
Ferr. *371.*

WRITER'S CRAMP
Cycl. *349*

X

XYPHOID
Kali bich. *454.*

Y

YELLOW FEVER
Crot. *336.* Carbo v. *213.*

YAWNING
Acon. *10.* Puls. *685.* Ver. alb. *855.*

WITH DYSPNOEA.
Brom. *139.*

FREQUENT YAWNING.
Bry. *150,* Caps. *204.* Caust. *230.* Kreos. *481.*

DROWSINESS, WITHOUT YAWNING.
Chel. *249.*

COMPLAINTS THAT COME ON WHENEVER ONE YAWNS.
Cina. *282.*

TREMBLING OF BODY WITH SHUDDERING WHEN YAWNING.
Cina. *283.*

VIOLENT AND SPASMODIC.
Rhus. *712.* Staph. *764.*

WITH STRETCHING AND EXTENDING HANDS,
Ruta. *721.*

Z

ZYGOMA
BONE FORMING BRIDGE BETWEEN TEMPORAL BONE WITH MALAR BONE.
Lach. *498.* Plat. *680.*

ZYMOTIC DISEASES
CHIEF FEVERS & CONTAGIOUS DISEASES.
Crot. *336/7.*

BIBLIOGRAPHY

Profuse references are made to 'Allen', 'Guernsey', 'Hering', 'Kent', 'Clarke' and of course 'Hahnemann' in nearly every chapter. As the actual books involved are not detailed each time, only books specifically mentioned are given in the following list:

ALLEN. Dr H. C.
Keynotes with nosodes. *3. 18. 53, 344, 483, 644, 689, 702, 830 835, 860.*
Materia Medica of the Nosodes. *488, 532, 689, 835.*
Keynotes of the leading remedies. *31, 52, 672, 731, 732.*

ALLEN. Dr T. F.
Encyclopaedia of Pure Materia Medica. *8, 27, 34, 67, 76, 77, 79, 111, 120, 174, 178, 183, 193, 249, 270, 282, 302, 310, 349, 387, 465, 535, 541, 602, 627, 640, 663, 669, 740, 769, 778, 781, 824, 845, 851.*

BOERICKE
Pocket book. *217.*
Materia Medica. *627, 726.*

BOERICKE & DEWEY
Edition of Schuessler's work. *379.*
Schuessler's twelve tissue remedies. *475, 523.*

BOGER. Dr. C. M.
Synoptic key. *379, 583, 770, 860, 867.*
Therapeutic key. *538.*

BORLAND. Dr. D.
Homoepathy for mother and infant. *215. 651.*

BURNETT. Dr J. C.
Diseases of the skin. *128.*
Change of life in women. *130.*
New cure for consumption. *830, 835.*
Organic diseases of women. *131.*
Fifty reasons for being a Homoepath. *151.*
Greater diseases of the liver. *346.*
Vaccinosis and Homoeoprophylaxis. *820.*
Diseases of the Spleen and their remedies. *231, 233.*

CLARKE. Dr J.
Dictionary. *17, 18, 82, 235, 276, 290, 310, 334, 339, 377, 418, 424, 453, 501, 537, 578, 587, 595, 617, 626, 662, 672, 695, 697, 700, 733, 817, 824, 832, 859, 867.*

COOPER. Dr
Cancer and cancer symptoms. *618.*

CULLEN. W.
Materia Medica. *252.*

CULPEPER.
Complete herbal. *244, 245, 363, 623, 770.*

DRYSDALE. Dr.
On pyrexin or Pyrogen, as a
Therapeutic agent. *688.*

DUNHAM.Dr. C.
Homoeopathy, the science of
Therapeutics. *548, 549.*

FARRINGTON, Dr E. A.
Comparative Materia
Medica. *180, 292, 652.*
Clinical Materia Medica. *124.
217. 304.*

GUERNSEY. Dr. H. N.
Keynotes. *12, 23, 43, 65, 72,
103, 305, 314, 342, 441, 540, 555,
629, 642, 673, 719, 770.*
Guiding symptoms. *249, 767.*

HAHNEMANN, Dr S.
Organon. *781, 853.*
Materia Medica Pura. *95, 106,
237, 320, 395, 403, 409, 536, 634,
760, 781.*
Chronic Diseases. *21, 41, 47,
132, 158, 320, 395, 432, 540, 546,
550, 551, 558, 662, 671.*
Conception of Chronic
Diseases as caused by
parasitic micro-organisms.
540.
Lesser writings. *851.*

HALE. Dr. E. M.
New remedies. *14. 111, 216,
231, 382, 648, 863.*
Diseases of the Spleen and
their remedies. *231.*

HALE WHITE. Dr.
Materia Medica of Pharmacy,
Pharmacology &
Therapeutics. *302, 330, 363,
464, 780.*

HANSON. Dr. O.
The Materia Medica and
therapeutics of rare
homoeopathic remedies. *624,
737, 797, 806.*

HERING,. Dr. C.
Guiding symptoms. *8. 59, 111,
165, 221, 270, 282, 284, 289, 302,
310, 337, 349, 375, 379, 387, 406,
422, 535, 541, 671, 740, 825, 835,
836, 851.*

HUGHES. Dr R.
Pharmacodynamics. *57, 178,
256, 270, 271, 274, 280, 284, 291,
387, 454, 522, 544, 639, 665, 725,
765, 768, 850.*

KENT. Dr. J. T.
Materia Medica. *85.*
Lectures on Materia Medica.
179, 396.
New remedies. *218, 805.*
Repertory. *626,*

MARCY. Dr. E. E.
Elements of a new Materia
Medica. *71.*

MINDERERUS.
Kriegs-Artzeney. *128.*

MURE.
Materia medica of the
Brazilian Empire, with
provings and the principle
animal and vegetable poisons.
339.

NASH. Dr.
Leaders. *583. 663. 737.*

NEATBY & STONEHAM.
Manual. *600.*

PARACELSUS
(Hohenheim)
Diseases of the Spleen. *231.*

ROBERTS. Dr. H. A.
Rheumatic remedies. *109.*

RUDDOCK.
Domestic Homoeopathy. *843.*

SCHROEDER Johan.
Pharmacopea Universalis.
128.

STORER. Christoph.
Medicina peregrinantium.
128.

TYLER. Dr. M. L.
Hahnemann's conception of
chronic diseases as caused by
parasitic micro-organisms.
Thuja. *825.*

WEIR. Sir John.
Homoeopathy – an
explanation of its principles.
7.
Present day article. *601.*

WHEELER. Dr. C. E.
Case for homoeopathy. *111*

British journal of Homoeopathy. *275,
286, 355, 456, 561, 850, 857.*
British Medical journal. *688.*
Cyclopedia of drug pathogenesy.
*101. 269, 330, 334, 349, 352, 437,
438, 462, 465, 598, 726, 758, 810,
858.*
Homoeopathic recorder. USA
1934. *18. 243, 806. 811. 834.*
Homoeopathic Physician. USA.
446. 690. 736. 803.
Hufeland's Journal.
(Hahnemann) *291.*
Stapf's archives. (Hahnemann)
21. 671, 781.